ONE MORE STEP

The 638 BEST QUOTES for the RUNNER

Motivation for the next step!

Selected, Compiled, and some even written by

Randy L. Thurman

iUniverse, Inc.
Bloomington

One More Step—The 638 Best Quotes for the Runner
Motivation for the next step!

iUniverse books may be ordered through booksellers or by contacting:

iUniverse
1663 Liberty Drive
Bloomington, IN 47403
www.iuniverse.com
1-800-Authors (1-800-288-4677)

Because of the dynamic nature of the Internet, any web addresses or links contained in this book may have changed since publication and may no longer be valid. The views expressed in this work are solely those of the author and do not necessarily reflect the views of the publisher, and the publisher hereby disclaims any responsibility for them.

Any people depicted in stock imagery provided by Thinkstock are models, and such images are being used for illustrative purposes only.

Certain stock imagery © Thinkstock.

ISBN: 978-1-4697-9319-1 (sc)
ISBN: 978-1-4697-9321-4 (e)

Library of Congress Control Number: 2012904487

Printed in the United States of America

iUniverse rev. date: 6/18/2012

Dedicated to race directors and volunteers
across the country.
You make a positive difference in people's
lives, including mine.
Thank you!

Introduction

On January 2, I weighed a "svelte" 205 pounds. My "executive" physical a few weeks earlier had been lots of fun. My doctor, trying to be humorous (doctors rarely are) told me I was *not* overweight—however, he informed me I was five inches *too short*. At five feet nine inches, I needed to lose forty pounds or more.

He "graciously" shared with me that I was in great shape—for a seventy-year-old. Unfortunately (or fortunately?) on February 18, I would turn fifty. He knew this of course, the wise guy.

So it was decision time. Should I continue down the path of "master couch potato"? Or should I do something about my physical fitness? The self-help audio book is telling me, "What goal would you set if you knew it was impossible to fail?" So I set a crazy, audacious goal: to lose forty pounds and run a marathon within the year—at age fifty. Crazy? Maybe.

The first friends I told reinforced just how crazy it was. "Don't you realize *how old you are*?" I didn't want to hear it. After my twenty-two mile run three weeks before the marathon, I finally shared the goal with close friends and family, and the response was the same. But by then I knew I could do it.

The toughest part, beyond starting, was staying motivated. I employed many mind tricks: I entered races, watched running DVDs, read running books, etc. What helped me most, besides entering races, was reading and memorizing motivational running quotes. Some were inspirational, some humorous, some simply "real." I mean, how can you read the following, by John "the Penguin" Bingham, and not be motivated?

> *The miracle isn't that I finished.*
> *The miracle is that I had the courage to start.*

Every time I read that quote, I want to get going, get started. I started collecting quotes from DVDs, books, and magazines. I searched the internet for running quotes. At racing events, I copied bumper sticker slogans and sayings on T-shirts:

> *I'm with the bomb squad.*
> *If you see me running, you'd better keep up.*

How can you not love that? I asked runners to share their quotes and wisdom (runners are like that). And every once in a while I would get a pearl of wisdom—such as when I asked a runner at the start of the race what his strategy was going to be. He responded:

> *"I plan on starting slow"*
> *(long pause, and then he grins ever-so-slightly),*
> *"then tapering off rapidly."*

How can you not smile? So I started to collect these quotes, bumper stickers, T-shirt slogans, and pearls of wisdom.

You have the best of that collection. These motivational quotes helped me on my eleven-month, marathon journey to take one more step (which I completed at the Route 66 Marathon in Tulsa, Oklahoma). I posted the quotes on my bathroom mirror and looked at them over and over while I was brushing my teeth or shaving. It makes a difference.

Happy running!

Randy

Why do I run?

Randy L. Thurman

I run for myself and for those who depend on me.

I run for those who can't and for great causes.

I run for those who can but need encouragement.

I run because someday I won't be able to, and

On that day, I hope and pray someone will run for me.

1

The miracle isn't that I finished. The miracle is that I had the courage to start.

> —John "The Penguin" (so-called, some say, because of the way he runs) Bingham, writer and speaker about running, after finishing a marathon when someone commented—after looking at him—that it was a miracle he had finished.

2

In running, it doesn't matter whether you come in first, in the middle of the pack, or last. You can say, "I have finished." There is a lot of satisfaction in that.

> —Fred Lebow, NYC Marathon cofounder, who ran the marathon of NYC's five boroughs two years after he was diagnosed with cancer.

3

Running is the greatest metaphor for life, because you get out of it what you put into it.

> —Oprah Winfrey, who successfully completed the Marine Corps Marathon in November 1994

4

To give anything less than your best is to sacrifice the gift.

> —Steve Prefontaine, who won 120 of the 153 races he ran during his career

5

The only reason I would take up jogging is so that I could hear heavy breathing again.

> —Erma Bombeck (1927–1996), an American humorist who wrote columns about being a suburban housewife

6

I always loved running … it was something you could do by yourself, and under your own power. You could go in any direction, fast or slow as you wanted, fighting the wind if you felt like it, seeking out new sights just on the strength of your feet and the courage of your lungs.

> —Jesse Owens, who broke several world records despite having fallen down a flight of stairs, and a year later became the first individual to win four Olympic track & field medals

7

The will to win means nothing without the will to prepare.

> —Juma Ikangaa, 1989 NYC Marathon winner (and winner of four other marathons) and successful trainer

8

Methinks that the moment my legs begin to move, my thoughts begin to flow.

> —Henry David Thoreau, American writer and philosopher, who made a habit of taking a four-hour walk every afternoon to get to know his neighbors and the world around him

9

A journey of a thousand miles must begin with a single step.

> —Lao-Tzu, Chinese philosopher who is commonly known as the father of Taoism

10

We run, not because we think it is doing us good, but because we enjoy it and cannot help ourselves.... The more restricted our society and work become, the more necessary it will be to find some outlet for this craving for freedom. No one can say, "You must not run faster than this, or jump higher than that." The human spirit is indomitable.

> —Sir Roger Bannister, first runner to run a sub-four-minute mile

11

Just say, "No thank you," and add, "I'm training for a four-hour marathon."

> —David Kuehls (contributing editor at *Runner's World* and a marathoner), on what to say to people offering you a dessert

12

You already have everything you need to be a long-distance athlete. It's mindset, not miles, that separates those who do from those who dream.

> —John Bingham and Jenny Hadfield,
> authors of *Running for Mortals*

13

Whatever you vividly imagine, ardently desire, sincerely believe and enthusiastically act upon … must inevitably come to pass.

> —Paul J. Meyer, who became a
> millionaire at age twenty-seven and is
> considered the founder of the modern
> personal development industry

14

You have to wonder at times what you're doing out there. Over the years, I've given myself a thousand reasons to keep running, but it always comes back to where it started. It comes down to self-satisfaction and a sense of achievement.

> —Steve "Pre" Prefontaine

15

Running is an unnatural act, except from enemies and to the bathroom.

> —Anonymous

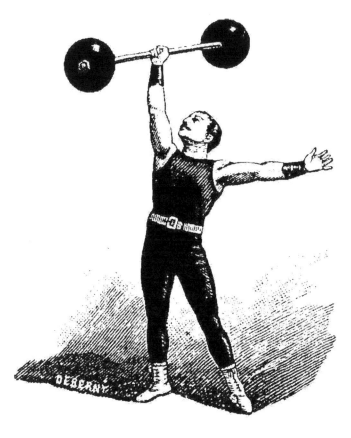

16

Running is a big question mark that's there each and every day. It asks you, "Are you going to be a wimp or are you going to be strong today?"

—Peter Maher, Irish-Canadian Olympian
and sub-2:12 marathoner

You also need to look back, not just at the people who are running behind you but especially at those who don't run and never will … those who run but don't race … those who started training for a race but didn't carry through … those who got to the starting line but didn't get to the finish line … those who once raced better than you but no longer run at all. You're still here. Take pride in wherever you finish. Look at all the people you've outlasted.

> —Joe Henderson, former chief editor of
> *Runner's World* magazine

Ask yourself, "Can I give more?" The answer is usually "Yes."

> —Paul Tergat, Kenyan professional
> marathoner, who held the world record
> in the marathon from 2003 to 2007

Whether you believe you can or believe you can't, you're probably right.

> —Henry Ford, American entrepreneur

20

I had as many doubts as anyone else. Standing on the starting line, we're all cowards.

—Alberto Salazar, three-time winner of the NYC Marathon

21

Racing teaches us to challenge ourselves. It teaches us to push beyond where we thought we could go. It helps us to find out what we are made of. This is what we do. This is what it's all about.

—Patti Sue Plumer, US Olympian who faced numerous physical challenges and setbacks yet continued racing

22

My doctor recently told me that jogging could add years to my life. I think he was right … I feel ten years older already.

—Milton Berle, American comedian and actor, supposedly after running a block

23

Running long and hard is an ideal antidepressant, since it's hard to run and feel sorry for yourself at the same time. Also, there are those hours of clear-headedness that follow a long run.

—Monte Davis, runner

24

Everyone who has run knows that its most important value is in removing tension and allowing a release from whatever other cares the day may bring.

—Jimmy Carter, US president and member of the US Naval Academy

25

18 Weeks ago … This seemed like a good idea.

—Back of a marathon runner's shirt

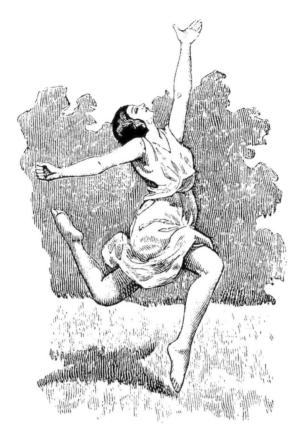

26

Play not only keeps us young but also maintains our perspective about the relative seriousness of things. Running is play, for even if we try hard to do well at it, it is a relief from everyday cares.

—Jim Fixx, author of *The Complete Book of Running*, who helped inspire the fitness revolution in America in the 1970s

27

Don't bother just to be better than your contemporaries or predecessors. Try to be better than yourself.

—William Faulkner, American author

28

Keep varying the program. Your body will tell you what to do.

—Joan Benoit Samuelson, first Olympic women's marathon champion

29

The difference between a jogger and a runner is an entry blank.

—Dr. George Sheehan, cardiologist and author of *Running and Being: the Total Experience*

30

What distinguishes those of us at the starting line from those of us on the couch is that we learn through running to take what the days give us, what our body will allow us, and what our will can tolerate.

—John "The Penguin" Bingham

Those who think they have not time for bodily exercise will sooner or later have to find time for illness.

> —Edward Stanley, Earl of Derby and British statesman, in "The Conduct of Life," an address at Liverpool College in 1873

Shoot for the moon. Even if you miss it you will land among the stars.

> —Les Brown, motivational speaker

There is an itch in runners.

> —Arnold Hano, author of *A Day in the Bleachers*

Perhaps BodyGlide™ would help.

> —A friend after reading the previous quote

It is better, I think, to begin easily and get your running to be smooth and relaxed and then to go faster and faster.

> —Henry Rono, Kenyan former athlete who, in 1978, broke four distance-- running world records in a span of just eighty-one days

35

I run because it's so symbolic of life. You have to drive yourself to overcome the obstacles. You might feel that you can't. But then you find your inner strength, and realize you're capable of so much more than you thought.

—Arthur Blank, successful businessman and runner

36

Anybody can be a runner. We were meant to move. We were meant to run. It's the easiest sport.

—Bill Rodgers, former American record holder in the marathon

37

No one ever drowned in sweat.

—Lou Holtz, American football coach

38

He who is not courageous enough to take risks will accomplish nothing in life.

—Muhammad Ali

39

The "Popeye syndrome": in a training program, there is no easy solution. Eating spinach won't get you through. You need to slowly but surely get fitter one day at a time.

—Jenny Hadfield, coach, author, motivational speaker

40

We may train or peak for a certain race, but running is a lifetime sport.

—Alberto Salazar, former American record holder in the 5000m and 10,000m

41

Spend at least some of your training time, and other parts of your day, concentrating on what you are doing in training and visualizing your success.

—Grete Waitz, Norwegian marathon runner, who won the NYC Marathon nine times—more than any other runner in history

42

Mental will is a muscle that needs exercise, just like the muscles of the body.

> —Lynn Jennings, world cross-country champion (in Mark Will-Weber's "Mind Over Matter" chapter from *The Quotable Runner*)

43

If you run, you are a runner. It doesn't matter how fast or how far. It doesn't matter if today is your first day or if you've been running for twenty years. There is no test to pass, no license to earn, no membership card to get. You just run.

> —John Bingham, author of *Courage to Start*

44

If you want to become the best runner you can be, start now. Don't spend the rest of your life wondering if you can do it.

> —Priscilla Welch,1987 NYC Marathon winner at age forty-two

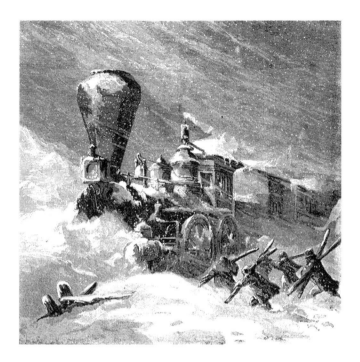

45

There's no such thing as bad weather, just soft people.

—Bill Bowerman, American track and
field coach and co-founder of Nike

46

To know you are one with what you are doing, to know
that you are a complete athlete, begins with believing
you are a runner.

—Dr. George Sheehan, cardiologist,
author, and a track star in college

47

We all have dreams. But in order to make dreams come into reality, it takes an awful lot of determination, dedication, self-discipline, and effort.

>—Jesse Owens, who won four gold
>   medals in the1936 summer Olympics in
>   Berlin, Germany

48

Same Day Finisher!

>—Back of runner's shirt

49

Mountains should be climbed with as little effort as possible and without desire. The reality of your own nature should determine the speed. If you become restless, speed up. If you become winded, slow down. You climb the mountain in an equilibrium between restlessness and exhaustion. Then, when you're no longer thinking ahead, each footstep isn't just a means to an end but a unique event in itself.

>—Robert Pirsig in *Zen and the Art of
>   Motorcycle Maintenance*

50

You can't delegate your exercise program.

>—Randy L. Thurman

51

The difference between a successful person and others is not a lack of strength, not a lack of knowledge, but rather in a lack of will.

> —Vincent T. Lombardi, American football coach (who the Super Bowl trophy is named after)

52

Pain is temporary. Quitting lasts forever.

> —Lance Armstrong, who won the Tour de France a record seven consecutive times

53

Adversity causes some men to break, and others to break records.

> —William Ward, American writer

54

Things that hurt, instruct.

> —Benjamin Franklin

55

Rules for Runners:
1. Have fun.
2. Be Kind.
3. Start slowly.
4. Run against traffic, mostly.
5. Look before you blow.

> —Bart Yasso, author of *My Life on the Run*

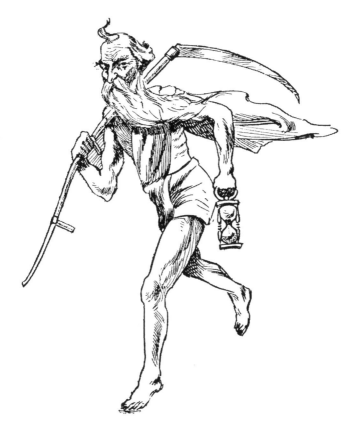

56

If you can read this, you were just passed by an Old
Dude.

> —Back of a shirt on a runner passing me
> in a 5k—I would guess he was about
> sixty-five

57

I hope I haven't missed dinner. I'm starved.

> —Charles Hardy, last finisher in the 1981
> Boston Marathon with a time of six
> hours, thirty-eight minutes.

58

I finished 837 in a field of 837, with a medical van and a motorcycle cop on my tail all the way. It made me feel like George Bush.

> —Rick Majerus, college basketball coach
> after losing one hundred pounds and
> running in his first marathon.

59

There's very little question now that I am a runner. How do I know that? I'm a runner because I run.

> —John Bingham, author of *No Need For
> Speed*

60

Many people shy away from hills. They make it easy on themselves, but that limits their improvement. The more you repeat something, the stronger you get.

> —Joe Catalano, a runner who reportedly
> likes hills

61

Why do I run? I run for my head first. Running provides me with a means to rid myself of stress. It is my "moving medication." No matter how I feel beforehand, I always feel dramatically better after a run. Running is simple. It costs nothing. You can do it almost anywhere. You can run alone or with friends. Simply put: running makes you look better, feel better, and live longer all at the same time.

—Tom Holland, *The Marathon Method*

62

There have been some race situations when I've had to go down to "one more step" to get me through a rough patch. This got me through.

—Jeff Galloway, who has completed more than one hundred marathons

63

You almost never regret the runs you do, you almost always regret the runs you skip.

—Mark Remy, author of the book *The Runner's Field Manual* (quote often attributed to Bart Yasso)

64

Running is a mental sport … and we're all insane!

—Unknown

65

Having a true faith is the most difficult thing in the world. Many will try to take it from you.

> —Steve "Pre" Prefontaine, who held the American record in seven distance events. He died in a car wreck at age twenty-four.

66

Running is a gift I give myself almost every day. Even on those days when things haven't gone great, I can come home and give myself the accomplishment of a thirty- or forty-minute run.

> —Arthur Blank, runner and businessman

67

My feeling is that any day I am too busy to run is a day that I am too busy.

> —John Bryant, *London Times* editor, 1994

68

There are clubs you can't belong to, neighborhoods you can't live in, schools you can't get into, but the roads are always open.

> —Nike ad

69

I cannot have survival as my only goal. That would be too boring. My goal is to come back in my best running form. It is good for me to have that goal; it will help me.

> —Ludmila Engquist (Olympic champion hurdler facing cancer and chemotherapy)

70

Commitment is what transforms a promise to reality.

> —Abraham Lincoln

71

I don't think jogging is healthy, especially morning jogging. If morning joggers knew how tempting they looked to morning motorists, they would stay home and do sit-ups.

> —Rita Rudner, American comedian

72

We are different, in essence, from other men. If you want to win something, run a hundred meters. If you want to experience something, run a marathon.

> —Emil Zatopek, 1952 Olympic gold medalist

73

I love running cross–country.... on a track, I feel like a hamster.

—Robin Williams

74

I'm never going to run this again.

—Grete Waitz after winning her first NYC Marathon. She later won eight more.

75

Man imposes his own limitations; don't set any!

—Anthony Bailey, writer

76

Vision without action is a daydream. Action without vision is a nightmare.

—Japanese proverb

77

What a moment of enlightenment it was to discover that there are individuals who are winning races irrespective of their finishing times.

—John Bingham, *The Courage to Start: A Guide to Living Your Life*

78

Some of the lessons to be learned about ourselves can be best learned as we push toward the edges of our abilities.

—John Bingham, *The Courage to Start: A Guide to Living Your Life*

79

Every morning in Africa a gazelle wakes up. It knows it must move faster than the lion or it will not survive. Every morning a lion wakes up and it knows it must move faster than the slowest gazelle or it will starve. It doesn't matter if you are the lion or the gazelle, when the sun comes up, you better be moving.

—Maurice Greene (often attributed to Roger Bannister shortly after running the first sub-four-mile)

80

Tough times don't last, but tough people do.

—Title of a book by Robert H. Schuller (later quoted by A. C. Green and others)

81

I run so my goals in life will continue to get bigger instead of my belly.

—Bill Kirby, swimmer and 2000 summer Olympic gold medal winner

82

I wanted no part of politics. And I wasn't in Berlin to compete against any one athlete. The purpose of the Olympics, anyway, was to do your best. As I'd learned long ago from Charles Riley, the only victory that counts is the one over yourself.

—Jesse Owens, who ran and won in the
   Berlin Olympics in front of Adolf Hitler

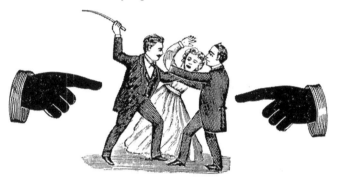

83

The ultimate measure of a man is not where he stands in moments of comfort and convenience, but where he stands at times of challenge and controversy.

—Martin Luther King Jr.

84

Once you're beat mentally, you might as well not even go to the starting line.

—Todd Williams, runner

85

Success is to be measured not so much by the position that one has reached in life as by the obstacles which he has overcome while trying to succeed.

—Booker T. Washington, American educator, author, orator, and political leader

86

Do a little more each day than you think you possibly can.

—Lowell Thomas, American writer and broadcaster

87

It is a rough road that leads to the heights of greatness.

— Lucius Annaeus Seneca, Roman Stoic philosopher and statesman

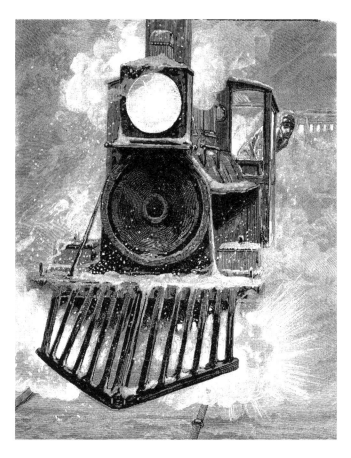

88

Even if you're on the right track, you'll get run over if you just sit there.

—Will Rogers, American humorist

89

Other people may not have high expectations of me, but I have high expectations for myself.

—Shannon Miller, seven-time Olympic medalist

90

If you run a hundred miles a week, you can eat anything you want. Why? Because

(a) you'll burn all the calories you consume;

(b) you deserve it; and

(c) you'll be injured soon and back on a restricted diet anyway.

—Don Kardong, American marathoner in the 1976 summer Olympic games

91

Ability is what you are capable of doing. Motivation determines what you do. Attitude determines how well you do it.

—Lou Holtz, American football coach and inspirational speaker

92

You have a choice. You can throw in the towel, or you can use it to wipe the sweat off your face.

—Gatorade ad

93

School cross country runs started because the rugby fields were flooded. There was an alternative: extra studying. This meant there were plenty of runners on sports afternoons.

> —Gordon Pirie, Olympic medalist and long-distance runner who broke five world records in his career

94

The five Ss of sports training are: Stamina, Speed, Strength, Skill, and Spirit. But the greatest of these is Spirit.

> —Ken Doherty, college track coach, from Mark Will-Weber's *The Quotable Runner*

95

The greatest pleasure in life, is doing the things people say we cannot do.

> —Walter Bagehot, English businessman and writer

96

Our greatest glory is not in never falling, but in rising every time we fall.

> —Confucius

97

Tomorrow is another day, and there will be another battle!

   —Sebastian Coe (a few minutes after
    a second-place finish in the 800m
    Olympic Games final in Moscow 1980;
    he later won the 1500m after having
    been favored to win the 800m)

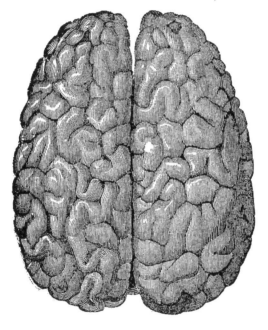

98

The nine inches right here; set it straight and you can beat anybody in the world.

   —Sebastian Coe (as he said this, Coe held
    his fingers up to his head)

99

Champions do not become champions when they win the event, but in the hours, weeks, months and years they spend preparing for it. The victorious performance itself is merely the demonstration of their championship character.

—T. Alan Armstrong

100

Real athletes run. Others just play games.

—Anonymous

101

In the absence of talent, there is no substitute for preparation.

—John Bingham and Jenny Hadfield, who have many, many quotes in this book

102

Running the marathon, for me, was accomplishing something that most people wouldn't even consider attempting.

—Randy L. Thurman

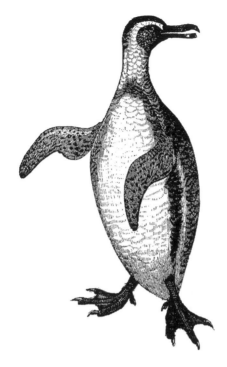

103

Finishing last in your first race is a sure-fire way to have lots to look forward to in your running career. I know: in my first race I finished just ahead of the ambulance.

—John "The Penguin" Bingham

104

How's my running? Call 1-800-eat-dust

—Back of a runner's shirt

105

Running is not, as it so often seems, only about what you did in your last race or about how many miles you ran last week. It is, in a much more important way, about community, about appreciating all the miles run by other runners too.

> —Richard O'Brien, English writer, actor

106

Because I'm good at it.

> —Frank Shorter, asked why he runs
> marathons

107

To get to the finish line, you'll have to try lots of different paths.

> —Amby Burfoot, American marathoner
> and winner of the 1968 Boston
> Marathon

108

Do what you can, with what you have, where you are.

> —Theodore Roosevelt

109

I know myself. If I ever get a headache, or feel ill or tired, I stop.

> —Lois Scheffelin, an eighty-plus-year-old
> runner

110

Through running we learn about succeeding and failing, about reaching past the probable, and accomplishing the impossible. The struggle to find one's potential as a runner is the most frustratingly satisfying pursuit many of us undertake.

—John Bingham and Jenny Hadfield in
Running for Mortals

111

My method of encouraging people to run is by running myself.

—Peggy Blount, runner

112

Running gives me confidence.

—Steve Prefontaine

113

Running gives you freedom. When you run, you can go at your own speed. You can go where you want to go, and think your own thoughts. Nobody has any claim on you.

—Nina Kuscik, Boston and NYC
Marathon winner

114

The true runner is a very fortunate person. He has found something in him that is just perfect.

—George Sheehan, doctor, runner, and
author of *Going the Distance*

115

I think there is too much emphasis placed on the distinction between people in the front and the people in the back. I happen to feel that the sensations are exactly the same for all of us.

—Kenny Moore, writer and marathoner

116

Running is real and relatively simple … but it ain't easy.

—Mark Will-Weber, editor of *The Quotable Runner*

117

It's not where you start—it's where you finish that counts.

—Zig Ziglar, motivational speaker

118

You are the way you are because that's the way you want to be. If you really wanted to be different, you would be in the process of changing right now.

—Fred Smith, founder of FedEx

119

If people are physically fit, they are better adjusted for life. Running is the greatest anodyne. It's mental therapy. While running, one develops a rhythm. The mind becomes detached.

> —Al Gordon, who was still running at one hundred years young

120

Some of us started running because nothing else eased the pain of living.

> —John Bingham and Jenny Hadfield, again.

121

There is no way to explain the feeling properly. It's one of those rare feelings that cannot be told to anyone who hasn't been there. It's simply the best feeling I've ever experienced.

> —Mark Osmun after finishing his first marathon

122

One of the most important factors is the ability to direct one's whole energies toward the fulfillment of a particular task.

> —Field Marshal Erwin Rommel

123

Every run is a great run!

—Sasha Azevedo, American actress, athlete, model

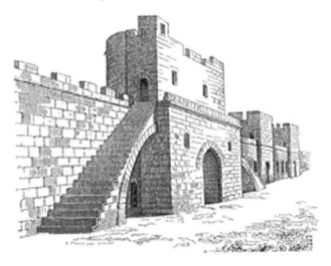

124

If one advances confidently in the direction of his dreams and endeavors to live the life which he has imagined, he will meet with a success unexpected in common hours. If you have built your castles in the air, your work need not be lost. That is where they should be. Now put the foundations under them.

—Henry David Thoreau

125

I've learned to read my body very well. By staying healthy I hope to run for the rest of my life. That's the big goal now.

> —Anne Audain, an Olympian and long-distance runner for New Zealand.

126

If all the benefits of running could be put into an easy-to-take pill, it would be prescribed more often than Viagra.

> —Randy L. Thurman

127

And on the seventh day, God did an easy three.

> —On the back of a runner's shirt

128

The only thing that's important in your training program is motivation. I've developed a set of motivational tricks that I'm constantly reviewing and refining. They have only one purpose: to keep me running.

> —Amby Burfoot, an editor at *Runner's World* for many years.

129

The true competitive runner, simmering in his own existential juices, endured his melancholia the only way he knew how; gently, together with those few others who also endured it, yet very much alone. He ran because it grounded him in basics. There was both life and death in it; it was unadulterated by media hype, trivial cares, and political meddling.

—John L. Parker, an American elite miler
and author of *Once a Runner*

130

Every run has the potential to transform us from who we are to the person we're becoming. Every step on every run could be the one that begins our metamorphosis from who we've always been to what we've always wanted to be.

—John Bingham and Jenny Hadfield,
Running for Mortals

131

Enjoy it, because you never know when it will be taken away.

—Michael Jordan

132

If individuals can get into the habit of starting workouts at a certain time every day, they will accept them as part of the regular daily schedule. Exercise will become habitual, and the day won't seem complete without it.

—Barry Franklin, exercise physiologist

133

I talk to myself when I train. The year I ran best at Boston, I focused on what to tell myself during those last few miles when it hurts. I told myself, "Keep going, you're a tough dude."

—Paul Thompson, runner

134

The right word spoken at the right time is as beautiful as gold apples in a silver bowl.

—Proverbs 25:11 (New Century Version)

135

You gotta hang in there. You don't know what is ahead. You don't realize what potential you have. You keep asking yourself, "Is it really worth it?" But you gotta hang in there.

—Brenda Morehead, Olympic runner

136

Great things are not done by impulse but by a series of small things brought together. And great things are not something accidental but must certainly be willed.

—Vincent van Gogh

137

I changed my belief from an external focus—beating others—to an internal focus. My self-worth was based on doing my best. I would compete only with myself.

—Henry Marsh, who represented America in four different Olympics in the steeplechase

138

He has to try running fast and slow, learn from his mistakes, and then figure out his own magic formula.

—Roger Bannister on how runners succeed

139

In running, it is man against himself, the cruelest of opponents. The other runners are not the real enemies. His adversary lies within him, in his ability with brain and heart to master himself and his emotions.

> —Glenn Cunningham, American miler in the '30s, who ran in spite of childhood burns that almost took his legs

140

We must search our limits of our body and demand that our spirit not give up on us.

> —John Bingham and Jenny Hadfield, authors of *Marathoning for Mortals*

141

There is only one big thing—desire. And before it, when it is big, all else is little.

> —Willa Cather, American writer

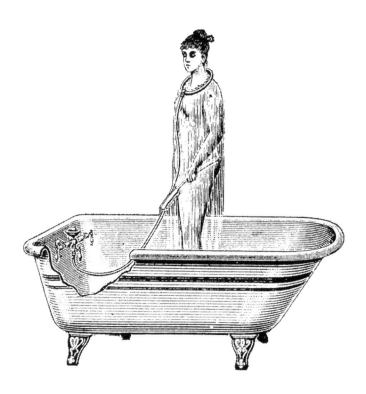

142

Think of taking a shower. That's just the point. It's so natural. It's the same with running. Just like a shower, running is part of my daily life.

—Nina Kuscik, winner of the Boston and
   NYC Marathon in the same year (1972)

143

Only two rules really count: never miss an opportunity to relieve yourself, and never miss a chance to rest your feet.

—Duke of Windsor

144

When you run in the morning, you gain time, in a sense. It's like stretching twenty-four hours into twenty-five. You may need to sleep less and get up earlier, but if you can get by that, running early seems to expand the day.

—Fred Lebow, NYC marathon director

145

You can succeed by finishing last.

—Joe Henderson, runner, and writer of more than twenty-five books

146

People ask why I run. I say, "If you have to ask, you will never understand." It is something only those select few know. Those who put themselves through pain but know, deep down, how good it really feels.

—Erin Leonard, runner

147

Running has never failed to give me great end results, and that's why I keep coming back for more!

—Sasha Azevedo, actress

148

Reality is for people who lack imagination.

—Bumper sticker

149

There are three goals in marathon running: to finish, to improve, and to win. Which goal you strive for depends on what level of running you're at.

—Hal Higdon, author of *Marathon: The Ultimate Training Guide*

150

Running teaches us to truly enjoy the moment—to find the happiness that eluded us in the past, the happiness that may not be there in the future—and to concentrate on living in this time of our lives.

—John Bingham, *An Accidental Athlete*

151

May your mind soar and your pants always fit.

—Unknown

152

It's clear to me now that I'll never have a runner's body, no matter how many miles I run. Instead I'm concentrating on having a runner's soul.

—John Bingham and Jenny Hadfield, *Running for Mortals*

153

Everything I see and feel is more extreme when I'm in training. If I'm happy, I'm happier. If I'm sad, I'm sadder. I once ran thirty-one miles, and after that there was nothing in the world I thought I couldn't do.

—Katherine Switzer, the first woman to officially enter the Boston Marathon

154

Each of us must have a mountain to climb, even if some might look on it as little more than a hill.

—George Sheehen, author of *Running to Win*

155

I run because I enjoy it—not always, but most of the time. I run because I've always run—not trained, but run.

—Amby Burfoot, runner and all-around great guy

156

All I can tell you is that because of running, my life is better. It is more fun, more productive, more meaningful, and I handle life's stresses better because I run. Running has given me more than I can ever give it.

—Randy L. Thurman

157

When it's pouring rain and you're bowling along through the wet, there's satisfaction in knowing you're out there and the others aren't.

—Peter Snell, great distance runner

158

Every time I bomb out, I have to come back. I have a feeling after a bad race that my next one will be good.

—Bill Rodgers, winner of the Boston Marathon

159

Most people who fail in their dreams fail not from lack of ability but from a lack of commitment.

—Zig Ziglar

160

Deciding to be a runner is only the first step. Actually being a runner is a daily commitment.

—John Bingham

161

You should run your first marathon for the right reasons, because you'll never be the same person again. You must *want* to do it, don't it because your boss did it or your spouse.

> —Bill Wenmark, running coach who has run more than a hundred marathons

162

There are as many ways to be successful as a distance runner as there are athletes. You have to develop a training schedule of your own.

> —Craig Virgin, world cross-country champion and Boston Marathon runner-up

163

A running machine that glides over mud, crud, and goop.

> —Ed Eyestone, two-time Olympic marathoner's definition of Kenyan runner John Ngugi

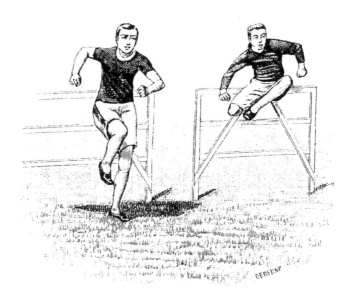

164

He cleared the hurdles like he feared they had spikcs imbedded on the top, and leaped the water hazard as if he thought crocodiles were swimming in it.

> —A description of Kenya's Amos
>   Biwotts's 8.51 steeplechase win in
>   Mexico City

165

Hold back for the first seven miles. Use it as a warm-up and then gradually increase your rate but never strain.

> —Adolph Gruber, long-distance runner on
>   how to run a marathon

166

My plan is to just wing it, and have a good time.

> —Mary Hearn, bike racer on her race
> strategy

167

I still love those long, easy runs on Sunday. They're the mainstay of any training program. It's like saving pennies: put them in a jar, and over a year you accumulate fifty or sixty dollars.

> —Robert Wallace, marathoner

168

Make running a habit. Set aside a time solely for running. Running is more fun if you don't have to rush through it.

> —Jim Fixx, author of the best-selling 1977
> book *The Complete Book of Running*

169

The motivation has to come from inside.

> —Martha Cooksay, American marathoner
> and former 15k record holder

170

Goals must be continually refined. Runners need to know the big picture, rather than just haphazardly go from race to race.

—Doug Renner, cross-country running
  coach

171

The hardest step for a runner to take is the first one out the door.

—Ron Clarke, world record marathon
  holder in the1960s

172

When people ask me why I run, I tell them there's not really a reason, it's just the adrenalin when you start, and the feeling when you cross that finish line, and knowing that you are a winner no matter what place you got.

—Courtney Parsons, runner

173

I'd phone in sick. I missed thirteen days in fourteen months and my boss finally sent me a letter pointing this out to me. Since taking up running, I've had only two sick days in the last fifteen months.

—Martin Kraft, runner

174

For most of my adult life, I was afraid of everything and everyone. As a runner, I learned that the fear outside of me was always overshadowed by the fear inside of me.

—John Bingham and Jenny Hadfield,
    Running for Mortals

175

Run into peace. The man who is in the state of running, of continuous running into peace, is a heavenly man. He continually runs and moves and seeks peace in running.

—Meister Eckhart, fourteenth-century
    philosopher

176

The first wealth is health.

—Ralph Waldo Emerson

177

Running is one of the best solutions to a clear mind.

—Sasha Azevedo, actress, model

178

People get a relief from tension by running. One thing that almost always happens is that your sense of self-worth improves. You accept yourself a little better.

—Ted Corbitt, former US marathoner and often called the father of long-distance running.

179

If you want to be successful in anything, it requires practice.

—Bill Wenmark, on running a marathon (who has run more than one hundred)

180

We arrive at where we are in our lives one day at a time.

—John Bingham, once an overweight couch potato with a glut of bad habits, including smoking and drinking; at age forty-three Bingham looked mid life in the face—and started running.

181

Be truly motivated to train for a marathon. Do it for yourself—not on a bet or a dare or because "everyone else does."

—Grete Waitz, marathon gold medal winner of the1983 World Championships

182

Running should be a lifelong activity. Approach it patiently and intelligently, and it will reward you for a long, long time.

—Michael Sargent, MD

183

Only he who does nothing makes a mistake.

—French proverb

184

There are two types of people. Those who run, and those who should.

—Nike ad

185

Success is the sum of small efforts—repeated day in and day out.

—Robert Collier, author of self-help books

186

Running is my sunshine. Every morning before I run, I say a prayer—giving thanks to God.

—Joan Twine, runner and running-shoe expert

187

If one can stick to the training throughout the many long years, then will power is no longer a problem. It's raining? That doesn't matter. I am tired? That's beside the point. It's simple that I have to.

—Emil Zatopek, Winner of the 5k, 10k, and marathon at the 1952 Olympics

188

I'd rather run a gutsy race, pushing myself all the way and lose, than run a conservative race only for a win.

—Alberto Salazar, 1981, 1982, and 1983 NYC Marathon winner

189

Don't let yourself be concerned by what other runners are doing. By trial and error, find out what works for you.

—Gayle S. Barron, 1978 Boston Marathon winner

190

If I get tired, I'll slack off exercising. I do get worn out. It's from the children, It's from work. I listen to my body, but I don't use that as a cop-out.

—Kim Alexis, model and runner

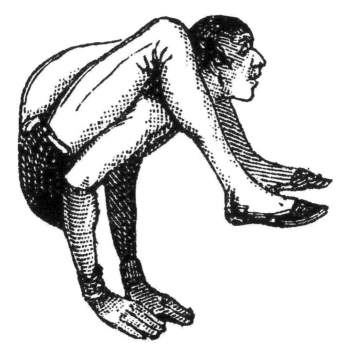

191

So much in life seems inflexible and unchangeable, and part of the joy of running and especially racing is the realization that improvement and progress can be achieved.

—Nancy Anderson, runner

192

Running is a statement to society. It is saying "no" to always being on call, to sacrifice our daily runs for others' needs. When we run, we are doing something for ourselves.

—Phoebe Jones, runner

193

My body immediately reacts to a lack of exercise. "Take me outside," it cries, "let me out."

—Paula Zahn, broadcaster and runner

194

My first understanding was that you could not become a distance runner quickly. I began gradually, not doing too much.

—Henry Rono, set world records in
the 3000m, 5000m, 10,000m, and
steeplechase.

195

I don't make a decision every morning. I made a decision once, long ago, to run every day. When I wake up, the decision is already made.

—Walt Guzzardi, who runs every day

196

The biggest tragedy in America is not the great waste of natural resources—though this is tragic; the biggest tragedy is the waste of human resources because the average person goes to his grave with his music still in him.

—Oliver Wendell Holmes

197

Friendships are born on the field of athletic strife and the real gold of competition. Awards become corroded, friends gather no dust.

> —Jesse Owens, winner of four gold
> medals in the Berlin Olympics; Hitler
> avoided acknowledging his victories
> and refused to shake his hand.

198

When you believe and think "I can," you activate your motivation, commitment, confidence, concentration, and excitement—all of which relate directly to achievement.

> —Dr. Jerry Lynch, sports psychologist

199

Anything is possible, but you have to believe and you have to fight.

> —Lance Armstrong, cancer survivor,
> who won the Tour de France seven
> consecutive times

200

Let him that would move the world first move himself.

> —Socrates

201

Somewhere around mile twenty, it hit me. Instead of a wall, I found the truth. At mile twenty I looked around and saw that not only was I with the "real" marathoners, but I was one of them. I was there. I was doing the miles. I was running at my absolute limit. Just like everyone else.

> —John Bingham, who started running at forty-three and has completed forty marathons and hundreds of 5k and 10k races.

202

Don't Pass Me … I'm not in your Age Group

> —On the back of a running shirt

203

Running is like mouthwash; if you can feel "the burn," it's working.

> —Brian Tackett, runner

204

The plain fact remains that men and women the world over possess amounts of resources that only exceptional individuals push to their extreme use. Compared to what we ought to be, we are only half awake.

> —William James, philosopher and professor at Harvard University

205

Rest is important part of a training program. There are times of the year when you should just go to the beach.

—Thom Hunt, distance runner

206

If people were possessed by reason, running marathons would not work. But we are not creatures of reason. We are creatures of passion.

—Noel Carroll, Irish middle-distance running star in the '60s

207

Take your mind, throw it up the mountain, and then follow it.

—Breast cancer survivor on how to achieve a hard goal

208

Don't think about how weak you are. Think of how strong you're going to be.

—Michelle (Berry) Dougherty

209

Yes, it was. But the harder I work, the luckier I get.

—Gary Player, pro golfer, after hitting a sand shot on the eighteenth hole to win a tournament and being told it was a lucky shot.

210

You didn't beat me. You merely finished in front of me.

—Hal Higdon, author of thirty-five books so far

211

There's always the feeling of getting stronger. I think that's what keeps me going.

—Frank Shorter, Olympic marathon gold medalist, 1972

212

Beyond the very extreme of fatigue and distress, we may find amounts of ease and power we never dreamed ourselves to own, strength never taxed at all because we never push through the obstruction.

—William James, philosopher

213

The best inspiration for a runner is to look at yourself naked in a full-length mirror.

—Michael Duty, runner

214

This is a magic moment for me. It's something I've been dreaming of all my life.

—Lameck Aguta of Kenya, after winning the Boston Marathon

215

I can still remember quite vividly a time when as a child I ran barefoot along damp firm sand by the seashore. It was an intense moment of discovery of a source of power and beauty that one previously hardly ever dreamt existed.

—Roger Bannister, first to break the four-minute mile

216

The idea that the harder you work, the better you're going to be is just garbage. The greatest improvement is made by the man or woman who works most intelligently.

—Bill Bowerman, Oregon track coach

217

What running did for me was, first, build my confidence and then help me come to grips with the unnecessary limitations under which I existed. My self-confidence has risen to a level where I can set goals that were previously unthinkable.

—Edward Epstein, runner

218

I've got the runs.

Bumper sticker on a runner's car

219

Running is the greatest thing that ever happened to me. It's the focus of my daily routine, the source of everything. It gives my life a sense of rhythm.

—Allan Ripp, runner

220

Run to Live,

Live to Run

—Bumper sticker

221

Running gives me a sense of controlling my life. I like the finiteness of runs, the fact that I have a clear beginning and end. I set a goal and I achieve it. A good run makes you feel sort of holy.

> —Nancy Gerstein, editor for the *New Yorker* (and a daily runner), when asked to describe her feelings about running

222

Successful marathoners must lose their cool, and allow this irrational, animal, consciousness to take over.

> —Bill Rodgers, four-time winner of the Boston Marathon and the NYC Marathon

223

If you are standing still, you're going backward.

> —Proverb

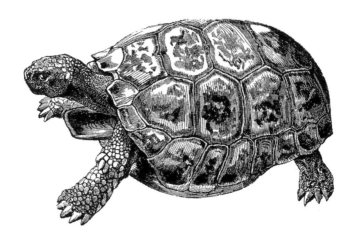

224

No matter how slow I run, I'm still faster than my couch.

—Anonymous

225

Some think "guts" is sprinting at the end of a race. But guts is what got you there to begin with. Guts start back in the hills with six miles to go and you're thinking of how you can get out of this race without anyone noticing. Guts begin when you still have forty minutes of torture left and you're already hurting more than you ever remember.

—Dr. George Sheehan, a truly
  inspirational writer on running

226

To finish a 5K in 23:59 is much faster than finishing it in 24:01.

—John Bingham

227

Jon says to Garfield "You know Garfield, running is 50 percent mental."

Garfield, still lying in his bed, thinks, *Pant, pant, pant, pant, sprint jog jog sweat sweat Phew!* And he then says, "I'll get around to the other half later."

—Description of a Garfield cartoon (drawn by Jim Davis)

228

The obsession with running is really an obsession with the potential for more and more life.

—George Sheehan, who ran a 4:47 mile at age fifty

229

I used to run to get to where I was going, but I never thought it would take me anywhere.

—Forrest Gump

230

When you hit the wall it hurts a lot, but then it doesn't get any worse.

—A runner's response to my question, "Does it hurt to run a marathon?" (Not quite the motivational answer I expected.)

231

If Found on the Ground, Please Drag Across Finish Line

—On the back of a runner's shirt at the Tulsa Route 66 Marathon

232

Stamina will get you there, but speed will get you there first.

—Peter Coe (1919–2008), father and athletics coach to Olympian Sebastian Coe

233

Everyone is an athlete. The only difference is that some of us are in training and some are not.

—Dr. George Sheehan (1918–1993); diagnosed with prostate cancer, he ran for seven years, making the most of every day

234

If you want to know your past, look into your present condition. If you want to know your future, look into your present actions.

—Buddhist proverb

235

Sustained motivation is essential to achieving your potential.

—Grete Waitz, Norweigian champion
runner who won nine NYC marathons
between 1978 and 1988.

236

I was unable to walk for a whole week after that, so much did the race take out of me. But it was the most pleasant exhaustion I have ever known.

—Emil Zatopek, describing his marathon
win in Helsinki

237

Bid me run, and I will strive with things impossible.

—William Shakespeare, *Julius Caesar*, Act
II, Scene 1

238

If I ever stopped running, I'd feel terrible, as if I were slowly decomposing. I enjoy being fit. There's a feeling of independence to it.

> —Bill Rodgers, who won his first Boston
> Marathon in 1975 with a time of
> 2:09:55

239

In my dictionary, the word "overtrain" falls just a page away from the word "overkill," defined as "to obliterate with more nuclear force than required." Consider the connection: if your target is top running performance, then to overtrain means to apply more force than is required to hit that target. In fact, overtraining may obliterate your target, or at least leave you without the will to pursue it.

> —Jack Daniels in Mark Will-Weber's
> "Training" chapter from *The Quotable
> Runner*

One chance is all you need.

> —Jesse Owens, seventh of eleven children
> in his family

What I am doing—nobody cares. It's personal satisfaction.

> —Kenny Moore, American marathoner,
> fourth place, 1972 Olympics

The secret of getting ahead is getting started. The secret of getting started is breaking your complex overwhelming tasks into small manageable tasks, and then starting on the first one.

> —Mark Twain (at times attributed to
> Agatha Christie)

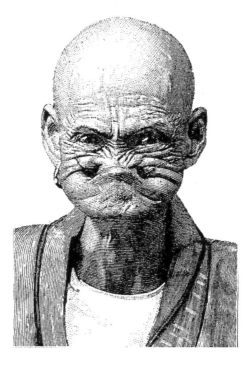

243

If you want to be healthy—run. If you want to be handsome—run. If you want to be smart—run.

—Ancient Greek aphorism

244

Very often a change of self is needed more than a change of scene.

—A. C. Benson, writer

245

If someone says "can't," that shows you what to do.

—John Cage, American composer

246

Running is a childish and primitive thing to do. That's its appeal, I think. You strip away all the chains of civilization. While you're running, you go back in history.

—Joe Henderson, writer and runner

247

For me, races are the celebration of my training.

—Dan Browne, 2007 national champion
in the 5K and 20K

248

Once you accept yourself as a hero, you can begin to understand that there are winners all along the race course.

—John Bingham, running advocate,
coach, writer

249

Success rests in having the courage and endurance, and above all, the will to become the person you are.

> —Dr. George Sheehan, whose books you should read

250

Every athlete has doubts. Elite runners in particular are insecure people. You need someone to affirm that what you are doing is right.

> —Lynn Jennings, bronze medalist in the 1992 Olympics and American 10k record holder.

251

The race is not always to the swift, but to those who keep on running.

> —Nike running poster

252

Some people follow their dreams, others hunt them down and beat them mercilessly into submission.

> —Neil Kendall, runner

253

Some people go through life standing at the excuse counter. Get out of line.

> —Ohio runner

254

Your body will argue that there is no justifiable reason to continue. Your only recourse is to call on your spirit, which fortunately, functions independently of logic.

—Tim Noakes, author of *Lore of Running*

255

Find your limits and exceed them.

—Lynn Strickland, runner

256

Afraid you haven't got what it takes? Then get it! Feed your mind.

—Ohio runner

257

Determine that the thing can and shall be done, and then we will find the way.

—Abraham Lincoln

258

If one could run without getting tired I don't think one would often want to do anything else.

—C. S. Lewis, *The Last Battle*

259

Self-conquest is the greatest of victories.

—Plato

260

The harder the conflict, the more glorious the triumph. What we obtain too cheap, we esteem too lightly; it is dearness only that gives everything its value. I love the man that can smile in trouble, that can gather strength from distress and grow brave by reflection.

—Thomas Paine

261

You must do the thing you think you cannot do.

—Eleanor Roosevelt

262

The body is given out on loan—don't waste it and expect to use it tomorrow.

—Shapiro

263

Act like a horse. Be dumb. Just run.

—Jumbo Elliot, pro football player, offensive tackle

264

The runner need not break four minutes in the mile or four hours in the marathon. It is only necessary that he runs and runs and sometimes suffers. Then one day he will wake up and discover that somewhere, along the way, he has begun to see the order and law and love and truth that makes men free.

—Dr. George Sheehan, running
philosopher

265

There are victories of the soul and spirit. Sometimes, even if you lose, you win.

—Elie Wiesel, Holocaust survivor and
author of fifty-seven books, including
Night

266

It's the quitting that really is hard.

—Gene Thibeault, who has run ultra-
marathons for twenty-plus years.

267

Heaven is under our feet as well as over our heads.

—David Thoreau

268

Above all, train hard, eat light, and avoid TV and people with negative attitudes.

—Scott Tinley, teacher, author, athlete

269

The body does not want you to do this. As you run, it tells you to stop but the mind must be strong. You always go too far for your body. You must handle the pain with strategy … it is not age; it is not diet. It is the will to succeed.

—Jacqueline Gareau, 1980 Boston
Marathon champ

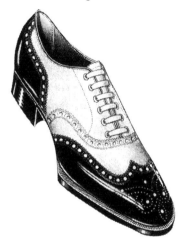

270

Remember the most important thing after choosing the right shoe is choosing the left one.

—Steve Jones, Chicago Marathon winner

271

"Sport" is not about being wrapped up in cotton wool. Sport is about adapting to the unexpected and being able to modify plans at the last minute. Sport, like all life, is about taking risks.

—Sir Roger Bannister, the inspiration for the movie *Four Minutes*

272

Bob does well in big races because he doesn't stand at the starting line and establish a pecking order. He doesn't look around and say, "Oh, so-and-so is here …" His great gift is his ability to focus completely on himself and his own race and then let the place or the time take care of itself.

—Coach Vince Lananna on Bob Kempainen, Olympic marathon runner.

273

I'm going to work so that it's a pure guts race at the end, and if it is, I am the only one who can win it.

—Steve Prefontaine

274

To a runner, a side stitch is like a car alarm. It signifies something is wrong, but you ignore it until it goes away.

—Unknown

275

You don't run against a bloody stopwatch, do you hear? A runner runs against himself, against the best that's in him. Not against a dead thing of wheels and pulleys. That's the way to be great, running against yourself. Against all the rotten mess in the world. Against God, if you're good enough.

> —Bill Persons, fictional coach in Hugh Atkinson's *The Games*

276

The trouble with jogging is that by the time you realize you're not in shape for it, it's too far to walk back

> —Franklin P. Jones, reporter, writer, humorist

277

I cried twice out there. It was beautiful. The people all along the way, standing there, cheering, yelling at you. I couldn't help myself. I cried twice.

> —Walt Ganty, on running the Boston Marathon

278

The only competition of a wise man is with himself.

> —Washington Allston, American poet and painter

279

It is better to wear out one's shoes than one's sheets.

—Genoese Proverb about work

280

Sweat cleanses from the inside. It comes from places a shower will never reach.

—Dr. George Sheehan, author of eight books on the running life

281

Endurance is patience concentrated.

—Thomas Carlyle

282

Fitness is a stage you pass through on the way to becoming a racer.

—Dr. George Sheehan

283

Obstacles are those frightful things you see when you take your eyes off the goals.

—Sydney Smith, English writer and clergyman

284

Human beings are made up of flesh and blood and a miracle fiber called "courage."

—General George Patton, old blood and guts

285

If a man coaches himself, then he has only himself to blame when he is beaten.

—Sir Roger Bannister, 1954 *Sports Illustrated* Sportsman of the Year

286

Some people run to get in shape … We get in shape to run!

—Front and back of a T-shirt

287

I chose to be an athlete. It is a simple choice, really, and one that you can make today.

—John Bingham, who, at age forty-three made a choice to run and is still running today

288

Those who do something and fail are infinitely better than those who try to do nothing and succeed.

—Lloyd Jones, author of *Mister Pip*

289

You comin' or not???

—On the back of a runner's shirt

290

The more I ran, the more I felt myself being freed from the shackles of a life of convenience, and the more I learned.

—John Bingham, who has more quotes in this book than any other person

291

Like each new day, each starting line is filled with potential. For a moment, only that moment counts. Each starting line holds the promise of greatness, even if that greatness is relative.

—John Bingham, see previous quote

292

It can be tempting to dwell on the total distance or on how far you are from the finish line. Try not to. Instead, focus on the mile you're running at that particular moment.

—Bart Yasso, inventor of the Yasso 800s and all-around good guy!

293

Sunshine is delicious,

Rain is refreshing,

Wind braces us up,

Snow is exhilarating,

There's really no such thing as bad weather,

Only different kinds of good weather.

> —John Ruskin, English poet

294

It's rude to count people as you pass them. Out loud.

> —Adidas ad

295

Rejoice, we conquer!

> —From *Pheidippides* by Robert Browning
> (allegedly his last words after running
> from Marathon to Athens to tell of the
> victory in battle)

296

Nothing gives one person so much advantage over another as to remain always cool and unruffled under all circumstances.

> —Thomas Jefferson

297

The only thing worse than running out of energy a mile from the finish line is finishing the race with energy left over.

—Bart Yasso, author of *My Life on the Run*

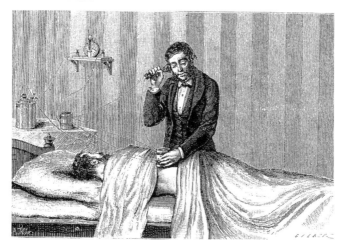

298

Listen to your body. Do not be a blind and deaf tenant.

—Dr. George Sheehan

299

For a time, at least, I was the most famous person in the entire world.

—Jesse Owens

300

Do or do not. There is no try.

—Yoda

301

There will be days I don't know if I can run a marathon. There will be a lifetime knowing that I have.

—Unknown

302

My sport is your sport's punishment.

—On the back of a runner's shirt

303

It's very hard in the beginning to understand that the whole idea is not to beat the other runners. Eventually you learn that the competition is against the little voice inside you that wants you to quit.

—George Sheehan

304

Don't fear moving slowly forward … fear standing still.

—Kathleen Harris

305

There is no satisfaction without a struggle first.

—Marty Liquori, third high schooler to break the four-minute mile

306

God has a purpose for me, and that is to serve him in China, but God also made me to run fast and when I run, I feel his pleasure.

—Eric Liddel in *Chariots of Fire*

307

Running is my medication when I'm down and my celebration when I'm up.

—Unknown

308

Mental toughness is only the confidence to go on when you can't move.

—Unknown

309

I run because I can. When I get tired, I remember those who can't run, what they'd give to have this simple gift I take for granted, and I run harder for them. I know they would do the same for me.

—Unknown

310

It is not the critic who counts; not the man who points out how the strong man stumbles, or where the doer of deeds could have done them better. The credit belongs to the man who is actually in the arena, whose face is marred by dust and sweat and blood; who strives valiantly; who errs, and comes short again and again, because there is no effort without error and shortcoming; but who docs actually strive to do the deeds; who knows the great enthusiasms, the great devotions; who spends himself in a worthy cause; who at the best knows in the end the triumph of high achievement, and who at the worst, if he fails, at least fails while daring greatly, so that his place shall never be with those cold and timid souls who know neither victory nor defeat.

—Theodore Roosevelt

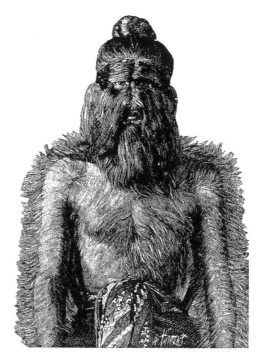

311

Wow, I didn't think you'd last that long by looking at you.

> —A tech administering my (Randy L.
> Thurman's) treadmill stress test

312

I thought you said this was 2.62 miles!

> —Back of a runner's shirt

313

To run and leap, to dart about with sweat pouring from your body, to expend your last ounce of energy and afterward to stand beneath a hot shower—how few things in life can give such enjoyment.

—Yukio Mishima, novelist

314

What do I get from running? Joy and pain, good health and injuries, exhilaration and despair, a feeling of accomplishment and waste. The sunrise and the sunset.

—Andy Burfoot, marathoner and writer

315

Set your goals high because what a person accomplishes is in proportion to what they attempt.

—Mitchell Naufell

316

I like finding out what my body can do.

—Charles Steinmetz, ultra-marathoner

317

I dream my painting and then paint my dream.

—Vincent van Gogh

318

All runners, at one time or another, are beginners.

—*The New York Road Runners Club
Complete Book of Running*

319

Start slowly and then taper off.

—Walt Stack, San Francisco running
legend (and also told to me at a race
regarding strategy)

320

I run because I want to. I run because through running I am discovering parts of myself that I didn't know were there. I run because most days it feels good to move my body with my own strength and will.

—John Bingham, who one day decided
to quit his bad habits and start running.
Now he is making a positive difference
in many lives, helping others run.

321

I've been running for more than twenty years. I read all the books and articles, yet I need a coach. Why? I still have to be told, to be encouraged.

—Fred Lebow, marathon runner and NYC
Marathon director

322

Give up TV and you'll be amazed at how much time you have to run.

—Kees Tuinzing, runner and publisher

323

Taking charge of your body can help you take charge of your life. And that power can help you go wherever you want to go, every single day.

—Cheryl Bridges Treworgy, member of five US world cross-country teams

324

The reason to run is to run.

—John Bingham (chcck out his website www.waddle-on.com)

325

A man too busy to take care of his health is like a mechanic too busy to take care of his tools.

—Spanish proverb

326

Running is a great investment. Your principal is low. Your rate of return is enormous, and it keeps growing every year. And there are no hidden charges, unless you count an occasional blister.

—Florence Griffith Joyner and Jon Hanc, *Running for Dummies*

327

The more I run, the more I want to run, and the more I live a life conditioned and influenced and fashioned by my running. And the more I run, the more certain I am that I am heading for my real goal: to become the person I am.

—Dr. George Sheehan

328

You have to be determined. You'll probably make great progress at first, but then you'll reach a plateau. You think you're going to stay there forever. When that happens, just be patient.

—Ian Pyka, shot putter on how athletes
   progress

329

I do better thinking when I run. If I'm stuck in the middle of a column, I'll go running and after a while it'll hit me. Either that, or a car will.

—Dave Barry, humorist and runner

330

Be yourself. You are the things you grew up with, the things your parents taught you. For years I tried to figure out who I was, where I came from. Now I feel it's important to be Dan O'Brien.

—Dan O'Brien, Olympic decathlete

331

Great dancers are not great because of their technique; they are great because of their passion.

—Martha Graham, choreographer and dancer

332

Work hard. Be dedicated. That's all.

—Charles Foster, hurdler, on the secret of success

333

To make life worth living, we must descend to a more profound and primitive level. The good of seeing, and smelling and tasting and daring and doing with one's body grows and grows.

—William James, philosopher

334

Running can be a way of discovering our larger selves. I am finding that average runners as well as superstars touch spiritual elements when they least expect it.

—Mike Spino, mind/body running coach. Founder of Run Into Spirit™

335

If you hear your inner voice saying, "What are you thinking? You're not a runner, you can't run," then I suggest you must run. And the voice inside will say, "Hmmm. You are a runner, you can run. What else can you do?"

—Randy L. Thurman, runner and compiler
of a really great running quote book

336

Long-distance running can give you a teenage cholesterol, remodel your lungs, lower your pressure, and slow your pulse.

—Dr. Richard Steiner, marathoner and
podiatrist

337

Each race is a new challenge. They're all different.

—Bill Rodgers, who held the winner's
medal of the Fukuoka Marathon,
New York Marathon and the Boston
Marathon at the same time. (The only
runner to do so.)

Most people never run far enough on their first wind to find out they've got a second. Give your dreams all you've got and you'll be amazed at the energy that comes out of you.

—William James, philosopher and
Harvard professor

339

The most important key to achieving great success is to decide upon your goal and launch, get started, take action, move.

—John Wooden, who won seven NCAA
national championships in a row as head
coach of UCLA

340

No matter how long you've been a runner, it is through racing that you learn the truth about integrity.... Before I raced, I was often tempted to both overestimate and underestimate my abilities. In life, as in those first races, I sometimes allowed myself to believe that I was better than I really was. More often, though I allowed myself to accept that I was much less than I really was.

—John Bingham (pick up one of his book
and get goin')

341

My other legs are Kenyan.

—Seen on a bumper sticker

342

When you first run up First Avenue in New York, if you don't get goose bumps, there's something wrong with you.

—Frank Shorter on the NYC Marathon

343

The quality of our expectations determines the quality of our actions.

—Andre Godin, philosopher

344

Courage is not the absence of fear but the mastery of it.

—Mark Twain

345

Performance wise, running in the adverse conditions helped, mentally it helped toughen us. Now they can see, they can do this. They have confidence now.

—Kim Williams, runner

346

Never go two days without running.

—Hal Higdon, runner and writer

347

Run hard, be strong, think big.

—Percy Cerutty, coach of Herb Elliott,
who set several world records and
pioneered "Stotan" resistance training

348

When I think I am too tired to run, I think of my friend Mark, who has been confined to a wheelchair since junior high because of a freak accident, and then I think of what a blessing it is to be able to walk and run. Then I get off my butt and enjoy the experience and thank God that I can.

—Randy L. Thurman

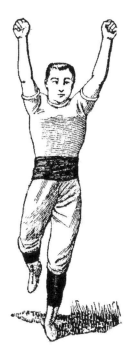

349

Now when I am asked why I run, the answer comes quickly. I run because through running I find answers to many of the other questions in my life.

—John Bingham, writer and runner

350

Do Not Pass!

—On the back of a runner's shirt

351

The answer to the big questions in running is the same as the answer to the big questions in life: do the best with what you've got.

> —Dr. George Sheehan (check out his
> website, www.georgesheehan.com—
> you'll be glad you did!)

352

Death is more universal than life: everyone dies but not everyone lives.

> —A. Sachs

353

He looked like a confused zombie, trying to sneeze while shuffling in concrete shoes.

> —A friend describing a runner (perhaps
> me) at mile twenty

354

You're doing great!

> —My friend Pat K, to me, at mile twenty
> of a marathon when I asked him to
> please shoot me and put me out of
> my misery. After those words of
> encouragement, I was good for the next
> 3.8 miles.

355

Not everyone who looks fast really is and not everyone who looks slow really is.

—Mark Remy, *The Runner's Rule Book*

356

One doughnut equals two miles.

—Mark Remy, *The Runner's Rule Book*

357

Have fun and finish.

—Best advice given to me about running my first marathon

358

Runners just do it—they run for the finish line even if someone else has reached it first.

—Nike ad

359

In the beginning you likely say, "I run." With more confidence, you say, "I am a runner."

—Gloria Averbuch, coauthor of *Run your First Marathon*

360

It happens to all of us, I think. The moment comes when what was impossible is possible, the unthinkable thinkable, the undoable done.

—Jenny Hadfield and John Bingham

361

You have to forget your last marathon before you try another. Your mind can't know what's coming.

—Frank Shorter, marathoner

362

Running is a thing worth doing not because of the future rewards it bestows, but because of how it feeds our bodies and minds and souls in the present.

—Kevin Nelson, *The Runner's Book of Daily Inspiration*

363

No matter our age or condition, there are still untapped possibilities within us and new beauty waiting to be born.

—The Reverend Dr. Dale Turner

364

Big occasions, and races which have been eagerly anticipated almost to the point of dread, are where great deeds can be accomplished.

—Jack Lovelock, 1936 Olympic champion
from New Zealand in the 1500m

365

I thought about how many preconceived prejudices would crumble when I trotted right along for twenty-six miles.

—Bobbi Gibb, first woman to finish the
Boston Marathon, 1966

366

No, I'm NOT on steroids. But thanks for asking.

—On the shirt of an extremely skinny
runner

367

It's probably the toughest distance race in the world to win. World-class runners from 1500m to the marathon contest it and instead of just three runners from each country, like in the Olympics or World Championships, in the senior men's race there are nine.

—Paul Tergat of Kenya, on the IAAF
World Cross Country Championships

368

There's no such thing as a bad carbohydrate.

—Don Kardong, author of *Thirty Phone Booths to Boston: Tales of a Wayward Runner*

369

When the meal was over we all had a quiet rest in our rooms, and I meditated on the race. This is the time when an athlete feels all alone in the big world. Opponents assume tremendous stature. Any runner who denies having fears, nerves, or some kind of disposition is a bad athlete or a liar.

—Gordon Pirie, 1956 Olympic silver medalist in the 5000 meters

370

I did it, I did it, I did it, I did it!

—A marathon finisher crying in the arms of a loved one at the finish line of the Route 66 Marathon

371

Get going. Get up and walk if you have to, but finish the damned race.

—Ron Hill to Jerome Drayton during the 1970 Boston Marathon

372

Motivation is what gets you started. Habit is what keeps you going.

>—Jim Ryun, former American athlete and
>   politician

373

It's easier to go down a hill than up it but the view is much better at the top.

>—Henry Ward Beecher, a prominent
>   clergyman, social reformer, Abolitionist,
>   and speaker in the late-nineteenth
>   century

374

Relish the bad training runs. Without them it's difficult to recognize, much less appreciate, the good ones.

>—Pat Teske, runner

375

I am too tired, even to be happy.

>—Gelindo Bordin, Italy, immediately after
>   winning the Olympic Marathon in Seoul

376

People who run find their lives so much more enjoyable. Everything works better: their cardiovascular system, their gastrointestinal system, even their ability to think.

> —Dr. Ralph Paffenbarger, runner and scientist

377

Physical fitness is not only one of the most important keys to a healthy body, it is the basis of dynamic and creative intellectual activity.

> —John F. Kennedy

378

It is not the mountain we conquer but ourselves.

> —Sir Edmund Hillary, first to conquer Mount Everest

379

It's a hill. Get over it.

> —Seen on the back of a runner's T-shirt (not Sir Edmund's)

380

Real success is failing to fail. Real success is looking honestly at what you can do, and then setting out to do more. Real success is knowing that failure is nothing more than a component of success.

> —John Bingham (you should know him by now)

381

Nobody's a natural. You work hard to get good and then work hard to get better.

> —Paul Coffey

382

God has given me the ability. The rest is up to me. Believe. Believe. Believe.

> —Billy Mills, from his diary entry days before his gold medal win in the 10k at the 1964 Olympics in Tokyo; he was the second Native American to ever win an Olympic gold medal, and the American who won gold in the Olympic 10k

383

Your biggest task is not to get ahead of others but to surpass yourself.

—Unknown

384

Keep away from people who try to belittle your ambitions; small people always do that—but the really great make you feel that you too are great.

—Mark Twain

385

There is no time to think about how much I hurt; there is only time to run.

—Ben Logsdon, runner

386

How does a kid from Coos Bay, with one leg longer than the other, win races? All my life people have been telling me, "You're too small, Pre," "You're not fast enough, Pre," "Give up your foolish dream, Steve." But they forgot something: I HAVE TO WIN.

—Steve Prefontaine (www.prefontainerun. com)

387

Success often comes to those who have the aptitude to see way down the road.

—Laing Burns Jr.

388

No matter what the level of ability, you have more potential than you can develop in a lifetime.

—James T. McCay, author of *The Management of Time*

389

I am both proud of and embarrassed by that run. What kind of geek goes out and runs in a cloudburst just before midnight on his honeymoon? Me, I guess. But probably many others too. You know who you are.

—Mark Will-Weber, *The Quotable Runner*

390

In a country where only men are encouraged, one must be one's own inspiration.

—Tegla Loroupe, Kenya,1994 NYC Marathon champion

391

You can't cram for a marathon.

—Bill Wenmark, running coach

392

Never give in, never give in, never, never, never, never
…

—Winston Churchill, from his famous
speech to the students at Harrow School
in 1941 (often quoted as, "Never, never,
never, never give up")

393

I was pushed by myself because I have my own rule,
and that is that every day I run faster and try harder.

—Wilson Kipketer, when asked if the
$50,000 prize tempted him to try to
break the world record

394

The new Kenyans. There are always new Kenyans.

—Noureddine Morceli, 1988, when asked
if he feared any other runners

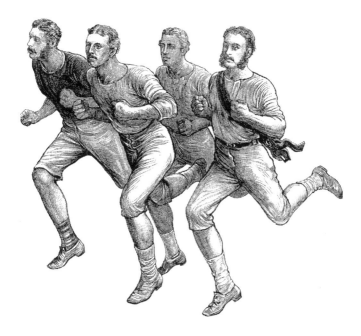

395

I run because it's my passion, and not just a sport. Every time I walk out the door, I know why I'm going where I'm going and I'm already focused on that special place where I find my peace and solitude. Running, to me, is more than just a physical exercise … it's a consistent reward for victory!

> —William Arthur Ward, author of
> *Fountains of Faith,* and one of
> America's most quoted writers of
> inspirational maxims

396

Dear God, please let there be someone behind me to read this.

—Back of a runner's shirt

397

I don't drink. I don't kiss girls. These things do an athlete in.

—Suleiman Nyambui, successful distance runner during the 1980s

398

The thinking must be done first, before the training begins.

—Peter Coe, in the "Coaches" chapter from Will-Weber's *The Quotable Runner*

399

To describe the agony of a marathon to someone who's never run it is like trying to explain color to someone who was born blind.

—Jerome Drayton, Canadian record holder in the marathon

400

Some runners may train to complete the distance within a certain time, but I wanted only to finish on the same day I started.

—John Bingham, on running his first
marathon.

401

Running is the classical road to self-consciousness, self-awareness and self-reliance. Independence is the outstanding characteristic of a runner. He learns the harsh reality of his physical and spiritual limitations when he runs. He learns that personal commitment, sacrifice and determination are his only means to betterment. Runners get promoted only through self-conquest.

—Noel Coward (1899–1973), English
playwright, composer, director, actor,
and singer

402

In short, running can change your entire outlook on life and make a new person out of you.

—Marc Bloom, *The Runner's Bible*

403

I'm with the bomb squad. If you see me running, try to keep up.

—Back of a runner's shirt

404

There is no finish line.

—Nike advertising slogan

405

Have a dream, make a plan, go for it. You'll get there, I promise.

—Zoe Koplowitz, Achilles Track Club member with multiple sclerosis, who required twenty-four hours on crutches to complete the 1993 NYC Marathon (from the "Victories and Defeats" chapter in Will-Weber's *The Quotable Runner*)

406

Great is victory, but the friendship of all is greater.

—Emil Zatopek, in the "Victories and Defeats" chapter from Will-Weber's *The Quotable Runner*)

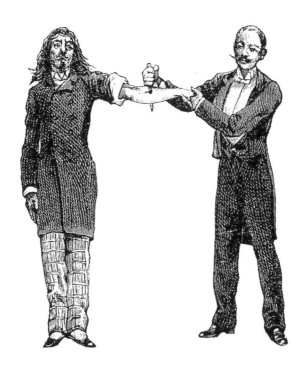

407

To keep from decaying, to be a winner, the athlete must accept pain ... not only accept it, but look for it, live with it, learn not to fear it.

>—Dr. George Sheehan, in the "Pain" chapter from Will-Weber's *The Quotable Runner*

408

I've had a wonderful time, and I made so many wonderful friends in the sport. I just like to run.

—Elaine Pedersen, one of the first women
to run in the Boston Marathon

409

Someone lent us a cottage in Hartfordshire. I was sitting in a sort of parlor there one day, writing. And suddenly I saw someone run past the window, along the lane outside. With shorts on, white shirt and so on. And it seemed to me such an unusual image... that I wrote down at the top of a sheet of paper, 'the loneliness of the long-distance runner.' I didn't know where he had come from, I didn't know where he was going. He was simply a sort of ... vision, floating by the window. And I put the line away, I thought I was going to write a poem with this sort of line in it. It seemed rather a nice line.

—Alan Sillitoe, author of *The Loneliness
of the Long-Distance Runner*

410

If you feel like eating, eat. Let your body tell you what it wants.

—Joan Benoit Samuelson, gold-medal
marathoner at the1984 Summer
Olympics

411

Talk to me not of time and place; I owe I'm happy in the chase.

> —Shakespeare, Epistle to David Garrick, Esq.

412

Men, today we die a little.

> —Emil Zatopek, on the starting line for the Olympic Marathon

413

Why couldn't Pheidippides have died here?

> —Frank Shorter's comment to Kenny Moore at the sixteen-mile mark in one of Shorter's first marathons (from the "Marathon" chapter in Will-Weber's *The Quotable Runner*)

414

Make your last thought before the start of a marathon: "If I'm not worried that I'm running a little too slow in the first half, then I'm probably running too fast."

> —Emil Zatopek, on the starting line for the Helsinki Olympic marathon

415

Running hills breaks up your rhythm and forces your muscles to adapt to different stresses. The result? You become a stronger runner.

—Eamonn Coughlin, in the "Hills"
chapter from Will-Weber's *The Quotable
Runner*

416

For optimum progress and peak performance, practice the three Ps of running: Patience, Perseverance, and a Plan.

—Jim "Jim2" Fortner, a legend on
Runners World Online forum

417

Every one of my runners is disabled in some way. For them, the race is a double challenge that many of them never imagined they could meet. Whatever they discover along the way has been inside them all along. What the marathon does is introduce them to themselves.

—Dick Traum, amputee and founder of
the Achilles Track Club, *A Victory for
Humanity*

418

Overtraining.

—Jack Daniels, coach of women's cross-country powerhouse Cortland State, about what type of training was currently popular among distance runners (from the "Training" chapter in Will-Weber's *The Quotable Runner*)

419

When you win, say nothing. When you lose, say less.

—Paul Brown, American football coach and team owner

420

Success in a marathon is running one step at a time, and doing that for 26.2 miles.

—John Bingham

421

Any idiot can train himself into the ground; the trick is working in training to get gradually stronger.

—Keith Brantley, marathoner (in the "Training" chapter from Will-Weber's *The Quotable Runner*)

422

Fear is the strongest driving force in competition. Not fear of one's opponent, but of the skill and high standard he represents; fear, too, of not acquitting oneself well. In the achievement of higher performances, of beating formidable rivals, the athlete defeats fear and conquers himself.

—Franz Stampfl, *Stampfl On Running*
(quoted in the "Fear" chapter from Will-Weber's *The Quotable Runner*)

423

I like running because it's a challenge. If you run hard, there's the pain and you've got to work your way through the pain. You know, lately it seems all you hear is, "Don't overdo it" and "Don't push yourself." Well, I think that's a lot of bull. If you push the human body, it will respond.

—Bob Clarke, Philadelphia Flyers' general manager, NHL Hall of Famer (from the "Voices From the Mid-pack" chapter in Will-Weber's *The Quotable Runner*)

424

A marathon is like life with its ups and downs, but once you've done it you feel that you can do anything.

—Unknown

I did the marathon because everyone said I couldn't.

—Jean Driscoll, eight-time winner of the
Boston Marathon, wheelchair division

We run because we like it, through the broad bright
land.

—C. H. Sorley, *Song of the Ungirt
Runners*

Don't quit, dammit!

—Marty Liquori, great American miler,
to Kip Keino during a 1972 race at
Villanova, when Kip wanted to back
out.

If the hill has its own name, then it's probably a pretty
tough hill.

—Marty Stern, coach of five NCAA cross-
country championships

429

Challenges are what make life interesting; overcoming them is what makes life meaningful.

—Joshua J. Marine

430

Some of the world's greatest feats were accomplished by people not smart enough to know they were impossible.

—Doug Larson, writer

431

If you want to tell something to an athlete, say it quickly and give no alternatives. This is a game of winning and losing. It is senseless to explain and explain.

—Paavo Nurmi, one of the famed "Flying Finns"

432

Apres moi le deluge ("After me the flood").

—Roger Bannister, after running history's first sub-4-minute mile. He was quoting Madame de Pompadour, though it is often mistakenly attributed to Louis XV, who said this after the French army was defeated by the Prussians in 1757

433

Concentration is the secret of strength.

—Ralph Waldo Emerson

434

Thanks, I've never passed anyone before!

—On the back of a runner's shirt

435

Yet that man is happy and poets sing of him who conquers with hand and swift foot and strength.

—Pindar, Greek poet, 500 BC

436

It's elevating and humbling at the same time. Running along a beach at sunrise with no other footprints in the sand, you realize the vastness of creation, your own insignificant space in the plan, how tiny you really are, your own creatureliness and how much you owe to the supreme body, the God that brought all this beauty and harmony into being.

—Sister Marion Irvine, 2:51 PR and 1984
US Olympic Marathon Trials qualifier

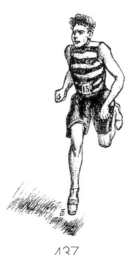

437

It is simply that we can all be good boys and wear our letter sweaters around and get our little degrees and find some nice girl to settle, you know, down with ... or we can blaze! Become legends in our own time, strike fear in the heart of mediocre talent everywhere! We can scald dogs, put records out of reach! Make the stands gasp as we blow into an unearthly kick from three hundred yards out! We can become God's own messengers delivering the dreaded scrolls! We can race black Satan himself till he wheezes fiery cinders down the back straightaway.... They'll speak our names in hushed tones, "Those guys are animals" they'll say! We can lay it on the line, bust a gut, show them a clean pair of heels. We can sprint the turn on a spring breeze and feel the winter leave our feet! We can, by God, let our demons loose and just wail on!

—Quenton Cassidy, fictional character in
Once a Runner by John L. Parker Jr.

438

Ask yourself, "Can I give more?" The answer is usually "Yes."

—Paul Tergat, who held the world record in the marathon from 2003–2007

439

Believe in yourself, know yourself, deny yourself, and be humble.

—John Treacy's four principles of training

440

The halfway point is mile twenty. Many, myself included, are convinced that there are usually eight and a half miles between mile markers twenty two and twenty three.

—John Bingham (believe it)

441

I am very determined and the sport is my passion. I believe I am born for running.

—Cathy Freeman, Olympic champion, 400 meters

442

Roger Bannister studied the four-minute mile the way Jonas Salk studied polio—with a view to eradicating.

—Jim Murray, *Los Angeles Times* columnist

443

My thoughts before a big race are usually pretty simple. I tell myself, "Get out of the blocks, run your race, stay relaxed. If you run your race, you'll win.… Channel your energy. Focus."

> —Carl Lewis, who won ten Olympic medals—nine gold

444

Maybe I shouldn't have had breakfast at Denny's.

> —Jordan Kent, who vomited after running the 400 meter in the 2002 USA Junior National Championships in Eugene, Oregon

445

If running were a drug, it'd be illegal: How great is it that we have access to this drug, pretty much any time we want, with unlimited refills? And that the side effects are almost entirely positive?

> —Mark Remy, runner and writer

446

Sure you have to know your capabilities. An untested, out of shape person should walk if he or she is feeling exhausted in practice or in a race. But the pain felt racing is the temporal price one has to pay for the ephemeral experience of a race well run.

> —Manciata in *Say it Ain't so Rage*

447

It's better to burn out than to fade away.

—Neil Young, from "Hey Hey, My My
(into the Black)"

448

I ran and ran every day, and I acquired a sense of determination, this sense of spirit that I would never, never give up, no matter what else happened.

—Wilma Rudolph, US track star

449

I definitely want to show how beautiful the marathon can be. I am the opponent of all those who find the marathon bad: the psychologists, the physiologists, the doubters. I make the marathon beautiful for myself and for others. That's why I'm here.

—Uta Pippig, first woman to win the
Boston Marathon three consecutive
times

450

Let's face it. Handicaps were made for golfers and bowlers. There's no reason to hold back and sandbag a 10k time. Despite press and media devoted to the contrary, running was never intended to feel good. Running is not a lifestyle choice. Simply put, it's a sport.

—Manciata, after reading the latest issue
of *Runner's World*

451

You find out by trial and error what the optimal level of training is. If I found I was training too hard, I would drop it back for a day or two. I didn't run for five days before the sub-four-minute mile.

—Sir Roger Bannister, the first to break
the four-minute-mile "barrier"

452

There will come a point in the race when you alone will need to decide. You will need to make a choice. Do you really want it? You will need to decide.

—Rolf Arands, writer, runner

453

Passion is pushing myself when there is no one else around—just me and the road.

—Ryan Shay, nine-time all-American
long-distance runner

454

When the guy says go, you start to suffer—or you might as well not be out there. It's a small piece of your life; make it hurt.

—Aaron Cox, winner of US mountain
biking championship

455

The trouble with a rat race is that even when you win, you're still a rat.

—Lily Tomlin, American actress and
comedian

456

Top results are reached only through pain. But eventually you like this pain. You'll find the more difficulties you have on the way, the more you will enjoy your success.

—Juha "the Cruel" Väätäinen

457

Your shoes are only as good as the laces they're attached to.

—Greg Sampson, former pro football player

458

Some people endure pain better than others. All things considered, the ability to withstand—or even deny— pain would seem to be a valuable ally for the long distance runner in search of significant improvement. In truth, it is probably a double-edged sword, since medical experts tell us that pain is the body's warning signal to back off, and that to ignore such schedules is to roll the dice with both body and mind.

—Mark Will-Weber, *The Quotable Runner*

459

Stadiums are for spectators. We runners have nature and that is much better.

—Juha "the Cruel" Väätäinen

460

Running teaches us that the only time we have is now.

—John Bingham

461

It's an incredible feeling, 110,000 people—energy at that level. What I realized from watching the first day of competition was that athletes that got excited and happy and got the fans into it and clapping, they did better. The athletes that took it too seriously, they didn't do as well as they'd hoped.

—Gabe Jennings, talking about his
Olympic 1500-meter semifinal

462

I feel the earth and the wind and the trees. I feel its spirit. It puts me in the moment. I feel the rhythm of the race. It's like music. When the rhythm gets dissonant and chaotic, it is either a jazzy driving force behind me or demons inside me.

—Gabe Jennings, about winning the 1500 meter in the
2000 Olympic trials

463

I took the lead. I wanted some people to run the real distance and that was frustrating. So I took the pace around the second lap, which in some ways is suicidal … but I wanted the pace to be honest.

—Marla Runyan commenting on the
women's 1500 meters at the Sydney
Olympics, in which she finished eighth.

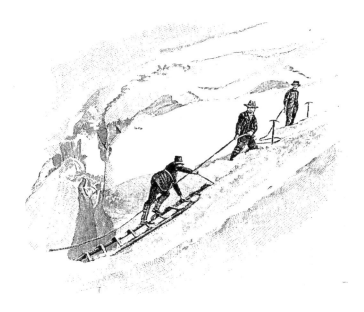

464

It is suicidal for other runners to copy my hill sessions without adequate background.

> —Pekka Vasala, Finnish middle-distance runner (who out-kicked Kip Keino at Munich Olympics in 1972, winning the 1500 meter in 3:36.3), about his legendary hill training

465

The mile has a classic symmetry.... It's a play in four acts.

> —John Landy, second man to break the four-minute mile

466

Chase after the truth like all hell and you'll free yourself, even though you never touch its coattails.

—Clarence Darrow

467

Tell the truth and run.

—Anonymous, Yugoslav Proverb (*Tell the Truth and Run* is also the title of a film about American journalist George Seldes)

468

Most men take the straight and narrow. A few take the road less traveled. I chose to cut through the woods.

—Unknown

469

Monitoring your body while training for a marathon is a little like teaching yourself how to write. You have to pay attention to what is being played out, listen to your instincts, make the subconscious conscious.

—Richard Harteis, *Marathon: A Story of Endurance and Friendship*

470

I ran for myself, not Finland.

—Paavo Nurmi

471

Inevitably, there's some official bellowing, "Come on! Run through the chute! Keep it movin' ... keep it movin'!" But you're bent over, gasping, admiring with salt-stung eyes the good, honest mud of battle, the trickle of blood from a spike wound, splattered on your still-quivering legs and too-old (but still lucky) racing shoes. What could be more beautiful?

—Description of the finish of a cross-country race from *The Quotable Runner*, edited by Mark Will-Weber

472

I want to be alone now.

—Honest feedback from an unknown runner reacting to another runner's attempt at encouragement.

473

The man who can drive himself further once the effort gets painful is the man who will win.

—Sir Roger Bannister

474

The mile has all the elements of a drama.

—Sir Roger Bannister

475

What was the secret, they wanted to know; in a thousand different ways they wanted to know *The Secret.* And not one of them was prepared, truly prepared to believe that it had not so much to do with chemicals and zippy mental tricks as with that most unprofound and sometimes heart-rending process of removing, molecule by molecule, the very tough rubber that comprised the bottoms of his training shoes. The Trial of Miles; Miles of Trials. How could they be expected to understand that?

—John L. Parker Jr., *Once a Runner*

476

Everyone in life is looking for a certain rush. Racing is where I get mine.

—John Trautmann, runner

477

The long run is the key. Skimp on weekly short runs but devote yourself to the long one.

—Leonard Davis, marathoner

478

I was totally into football, totally into mainstream sports my whole life.... The media has tried to categorize me, call me a hippie, call me alternative. I work hard. My social life and beliefs don't get in the way of my training.

—Gabe Jennings, who gave up football
his freshman year, becoming one of
America's best high-school milers

479

Even if you fall flat on your face, at least you are moving forward.

—Sue Luke

480

Our battles are not for position or for awards. Our battles are most often not even with one another. All of us have come to this place and donned our armor to face our most brutal enemy—ourselves.

—John Bingham

481

Pain is temporary; pride is forever!

—Anonymous

482

I am in a world of pain, but I'm happy. I survived the water obstacle, and I can't even swim.

—Briton Mark Hawkins, finisher from Bristol, in the 2002 Wife-Carrying World Championships

483

You only get to negatively affect your DNA.

—Manciata's explanation for why some people can't run a marathon

484

No doubt a brain and some shoes are essential for marathon success, although if it comes down to a choice, pick the shoes. More people finish marathons with no brains than with no shoes.

—Don Kardong, president of the Road Runners Club of America from 1996–2000

485

[Scientific testing] can't determine how the mind will tolerate pain in a race. Sometimes, I say, "Today I can die."

—Gelindo Bordin, winner of the 1988
  Olympic marathon

486

That is the sort of race which one really enjoys—to feel at one's peak on the day when it is necessary, and to be able to produce the pace at the very finish. It gives a thrill which compensates for months of training and toiling. But it is the sort of race that one wants only about once a season.

—Jack Lovelock, held world mile record
  in 1933 at 4:07.6

487

Nothing splendid has ever been achieved except by those who dared believe that something inside them was superior to circumstance.

—Bruce Barton (1886–1967), American
  author, advertising executive, and
  politician

488

Runners are the Don Quixotes of the world, forever flailing at windmills, sometimes laughed at, rarely understood.

> —Michael Sandrock, author of *Running Tough*

489

The trouble with jogging is that the ice falls out of your glass.

> —Martin Mull, American comedian

490

The idea of losing the three at Hayward Field and the idea of losing my specialty to someone who wasn't running his specialty. Mostly, the idea of losing in front of my people. They haven't forgotten about me.

> —Steve Prefontaine, when asked by a reporter how he mustered enough strength on the last two hundred yards to catch Frank Shorter by six tenths of a second and establish a new American three-mile record at 12:51.4.

491

It is amazing how much you can progress week after week, month after month, year after year if you allow for gradual training increases.

—Bob Glover, *The Runner's Handbook*

492

Out on the roads there is fitness and self-discovery and the persons we were destined to be.

—Dr. George Sheehan

493

There are as many reasons for running as there are days in the year, years in my life. But mostly I run because I am an animal and a child, an artist and a saint. So, too, are you. Find your own play, your own self-renewing compulsion, and you will become the person you are meant to be.

—Dr. George Sheehan

494

A good hill definitely levels the playing field for a lot of runners, which means more of us not only will run closer together, but we will get a quality workout that would not be the same otherwise.

—The Rage, on *Beating Your Buddies*

495

I want to run with the Kenyans ... Where'd they go?

   —Front and back of a running T-shirt

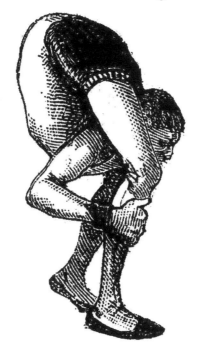

496

Hard things take time to do. Impossible things just take a little longer.

      —Percy Cerutty, one of the world's
         leading running coaches in the 1950s
         and 1960s

497

Most of us don't wear out—we rust.

—An anonymous physician

498

I felt my throat start to close up, and I didn't think I was getting enough oxygen. I was scared, and I thought about quitting. But you don't want to quit when you've trained so hard and long for one race.

—Deena Drossin, describing the effects of having been stung by a bee in the back of the throat one hundred meters after the start of the World Cross-Country Championships in Portugal. Despite blacking out and falling down during the 8k race, she finished in twelfth place.

499

It came like electricity, it came from every fiber, from his fingertips to his toes. It came as a broad waters come through a gorge. He called on it all.

—Norman Harris, description of Jack Lovelock's finishing kick to win the 1936 Olympic 1500

500

The time of your life is often as simple as giving in to the joy of the moment.

>—John Bingham

501

I just run as hard as I can for twenty miles and then race.

>—Steve Jones (when he was asked about his race plan after he had won the Chicago Marathon in the world's best time)

502

Anyone can run twenty miles. It's the next six that count.

>—Barry Magee, marathon bronze in Rome, 1960

503

Hills are speedwork in disguise.

>—Frank Shorter, who won the gold medal in the 1972 Munich Olympic marathon, silver medal in the 1976 Montreal Olympics

504

My legs aching, my chest aching, my heart thumping and banging away, the only things to look forward to, the only things that kept me going, the drinks of water; but only when he offered them, I'd never ask for them, no matter how I felt, any more than I'd stop till the old bastard said I could stop. Except twice to be sick, while he just stood watching me while it all came heaving out, not saying anything; just standing, waiting for me to go on, while I thought Christ I'll die, I'm going to die, my guts are coming out, I'll die.

—Ike Low, miler in *The Olympian*

505

Mind is everything: muscle—pieces of rubber. All that I am, I am because of my mind.

—Paavo Nurmi, set world records in the 1500m and the 20km in the 1920s

506

The things we do should consume us. If they don't, our lives won't have any meaning.

—John J. Kelley, 1957 Boston Marathon winner

507

Begin at the beginning and go on till you come to the end; then stop.

> —The King, from *Alice in Wonderland* by
> Lewis Carroll

508

A miler's kick does the trick ... a miler's kick does the trick.

> —Rod Dixon's mental refrain as he chased
> down and beat Geoff Smith in the last
> half mile of the 1983 NYC Marathon.
> Dixon won bronze in the 1500 at the
> Munich Olympics.

509

Thank God it's over.

> —Neil Cusack, 1974 marathon winner

510

You make it all sound so simple. Run your guts out … collapse at the finish, throw up, that makes a good runner. Sounds like you regret not being more like Prefontaine.… Everyone gripes to me that American marathoners are "lazy-no-good-for-nothings." My point is, many people have criticisms, but few have valid answers. I'd like to know what happened to the guys who kicked my ass in high school.

—Keith Brantly, in response to John
Shieffer's criticism of American
distance runners

511

No one competes with the reckless abandon they should. What is a race? A racc is a complete all out effort. With a few exceptions, runners run hard, (or think they are running hard) but the races are too controlled. When was the last time you saw an American distance runner finish a race and then collapse on the ground? Ten, fifteen years? I'd personally rather watch someone who runs his guts out, throws his breakfast up and passes out at the end of the race.

—John Schiefer, NCAA All-American
1500m

512

Americans have not had the same successes because of the fact that most grow up in the lap of luxury. They don't tolerate the type of pain that distance running demands. You can pass your physical education classes in school by walking a mile maybe twice a year. It seems that the few Americans who do make it on the international level have a tremendous drive and tolerance for discomfort. I think the main reason Africans succeed in distance running is many have to and we don't.

—Ryan Wilson, who has one of the fastest times ever in the 110m hurdles.

513

I have been wearied by the misrepresentation of my sport by the national and local media.... It reminds me of a scene in the movie *Educating Rita*, where the old mother half-cries during a rather mechanized group sing-a-long at a local pub, "Doesn't anyone know another song?"

—Joan Nesbit, full-time mommy, part-time coach, sideline runner

514

Many statistics say we only use a small percentage of our brains. I think the same can be said about our body.

—Peter Martins and the New York City Ballet, *New York City Ballet Workout*

515

After I left the podium in Atlanta, I felt so fulfilled in my career that I lost my desire to compete at that level again.

> —Carl Lewis, after the Atlanta Olympics
> and winning his ninth gold medal

516

Worry about him? I never even heard of him.

> —Ron Clarke, Australian distance runner,
> on Billy Mills' 10,000m victory in the
> Tokyo Olympics, 1964

517

Coming off the last turn, my thoughts changed from, *One more try, one more try, one more try ...* to *I can win! I can win! I can win!*

> —Billy Mills, who beat Clarke in Tokyo

518

I wanted to run my race. I didn't want to sit there and play games and see who could kick the hardest. I wanted it to be a race.

> —Marla Runyan, a legally blind marathon
> runner, 2:32:15

519

I'm going to go and leave my blood all over the track.

> —Nick Rogers, Olympian who at the trials
> finished third in the 5000m taking the
> race away from the kickers by grabbing
> the lead with a mile to go and forcing
> the pace

520

The victory of each run, the victory of each race, has nothing to do with winning or losing. It has nothing to do with finishing a run or a race that truly shouldn't be finished. It has to do with learning how to be who you honestly are, at every moment.

> —John Bingham

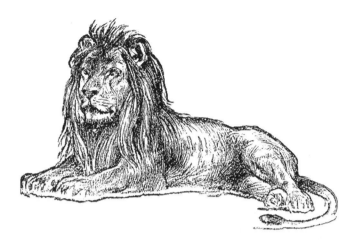

521

It's the road signs: "Beware of lions."

—Kip Lagat, Kenyan distance runner, explaining during the Sydney Olympics why his country produces so many great runners

522

If you can't win, make the fellow ahead of you break the record.

—Unknown

523

When the gun shoots, you got to go.

—Ato Boldon, four-time Olympic medal winner

524

I made the school team, and when I won in a match against another school it was the greatest moment of my life—even greater than the European titles. In those school races, I always ran my legs off. There were girls watching and I wanted to impress them. I was foaming and vomiting, but I won.

> —Juha Väätäinen of Finland, who
> won gold in the 1971 European
> Championships in the 5000m and the
> 10,000m

525

Running on an artificial leg at full speed is like driving backward at fifty-five miles per hour, using only your rear-view mirror to guide you.

> —Thomas Bourgeois, Paralympic athlete
> from America who competes mainly in
> category P44 pentathlon events.

526

I haven't seen too many American distance men on the international scene willing to take risks. I saw some US women in Barcelona willing to risk, more than men. The Kenyans risk. I risked—I went through the first half of the Tokyo race just a second off my best 5000 time.

> —Billy Mills, gold-medal winner of the
> 10,000 at the 1964 Tokyo Olympics with
> a personal record (PR) by 46 seconds

527

Strong people are made by opposition, like kites that go up against the wind.

—Frank Harris (1856–1931), author,
editor, journalist, publisher

528

To succeed, you have to believe in something with such a passion that it becomes a reality.

—Anita Roddick, founder of The Body
Shop

529

The perfect run? The wind at your back, the sun in front of you, and your friends by your side.

—Aaron Douglas Trimble, marathoner

530

Strong lives are motivated by dynamic purposes.

—Kenneth Hildebrand, author of
Achieving Real Happiness

531

The clock isn't slower; you're just faster.

—Adidas

532

It doesn't matter how slow you go, as long as you do not stop.

> —Confucius

533

If I am still standing at the end of the race, hit me with a board and knock me down, because that means I didn't run hard enough.

> —Steve Jones, former world marathon
> record holder

534

Few of us know what we are capable of doing ... we have never pushed ourselves hard enough to find out.

> —Alfred A. Montapert, author of *The
> Supreme Philosophy of Man: The Laws
> of Life*

535

This is where you will win the battle—in the playhouse of your mind.

> —Maxwell Maltz, author of *Psycho-
> Cybernetics*

536

I started running at age seventy-two because I was tired of all the boring talk about funerals.

—Ruth Rothfarb, marathon runner at age eighty-one

537

The task ahead of you is never greater than the strength within you.

—Unknown

538

Aspire to be great instead of good, aspire to be remembered instead of forgotten, aspire to accomplish what others have and have not done, aspire to be yourself and nothing else for when you strive to be yourself everything is limitless because you are not holding yourself to the limits of others.

—Troy Streacker, runner

539

I run, therefore I am. I am, when I run.

—Randy L. Thurman

540

Hunker down, keep your eyes fixed ahead, and run like hell.

—Paul Spangler, advice to Sister Marion before a race.

541

You must realize one thing. In every little village in the world there are great potential champions who only need motivation, development, and good exercise evaluation.

—Arthur Lydiard, New Zealand runner
and coach

542

Intelligent coaching is sometimes no coaching.

—Marty Stern, women's cross-country
coaching legend

543

My greatest ideas stem from running.

—Sasha Azevedo, American actress,
athlete, model

544

My favorite moments are when I pass someone who's huffing and puffing and all I got are some slightly tired legs.

—Troy Streacker, runner

545

Q. Why aren't you signed up for the 401K?

A. I'd never be able to run that far.

—Scott Adams, "Dilbert" (4/2/01)

546

Heart is the difference between those who *attempt* and those who *achieve*.

—Anonymous

547

We are what we repeatedly do. Excellence, then, is not an act but a habit.

—Aristotle

548

Pain is temporary; finishing is forever.

—Anonymous

549

It takes a little more persistence to get up and go the distance.

—Song lyric from "The Enemy Within (Part One of Fear)" by Rush (written by Neil Peart)

550

The marathon can humble you.

—Bill Rodgers

551

At my school, I was timekeeper. It was my responsibility to make sure the other students were on time. So it was important that I arrived always first.

> —Ibraham Hussein on running miles to
> school as a child in Kenya

552

An object at rest tends to stay at rest and an object in motion tends to stay in motion.

> —Sir Isaac Newton, Newton's First Law
> of Motion

553

Man, lose no time, get up, and take the course again, for he who rises again quickly and continues the race is as if never fallen.

> —Molinos, founder of Quietude (and
> quoted by William James in *The Variety
> of Religious Experience*)

554

Last is just the slowest winner.

> —C. Hunter Boyd

555

Anybody running beats anybody walking, and anybody walking beats anybody sitting.

—Tom Bunk

556

It's not 13.1 miles … it's seven water stops.

—Anonymous

557

I've never been beaten by the guy behind me.

—Anonymous

558

Pain is weakness leaving your body.

—Marine Corps (also attributed to Nietzsche)

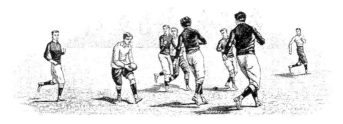

559

If it were any easier, they might call it football.

—Anonymous

560

Pain is nothing compared to what it feels like to quit.

>—Anonymous

561

Follow me—I know the way

>—Herman Cohen, as he led a large group
>astray at the Nugget 100 miler, 1994

562

If you think you won't finish, you won't.

>—Dick Collins, a runner in his sixties,
>who ran hundreds of marathons and
>ultra-marathons

563

Only those who will risk going too far can possibly find out how far they can go.

>—T. S. Eliot

564

Great spirits often encounter violent opposition from mediocre minds.

>—Albert Einstein

565

If you can't fly, then run. If you can't run, then walk. If you can't walk, then crawl. But whatever you do, keep moving.

—Martin Luther King Jr.

566

The endurance athlete is the ultimate realist.

—Marty Liquori, who made the US Olympic team at nineteen years old

567

Fatigue makes cowards of us all.

—Vince Lombardi, quoting Gen. George S. Patton (the second half of the quote is, "Men in condition do not tire")

568

Champions are born with the right stuff but still must suffer the stresses of training to achieve full potential.

—David Costill, a pioneer in the study of exercise science and performance maximization, who studied different types of muscle fibers and why some runners excel at sprinting while others are better at endurance races

569

The purpose of training is to stress the body, so when you rest it will grow stronger and more tolerant of the demands of distant running.

  —David Costill

570

The most important thing in life is not the triumph but the struggle. The essential thing is not to have conquered but to have fought well.

  —Pierre de Courbertin, considered the
   father of the modern Olympic games

571

The road to excess leads to the place of wisdom, for we can never know what is enough until we have experienced too much.

  —William Blake, English poet, painter,
   and printmaker

572

Succeeding makes you forget the failures.

  —Harry Cordellos, blind athlete who
   finished 2:57 at Boston in 1975

573

Nothing ever fatigues me, except that which I dislike.

—Jane Austen, English novelist

574

Runners can get through the weary and lonely hours only if they are at peace themselves.

—Ayers, runner

575

If you under-train, you may not finish, but if you overtrain, you may not start.

—Tom DuBos, runner

576

There ain't no shame looking at a good runner's back. Now, if the runner sucks, that's something else entirely.

—The Rage, in *Training Tips "Comeback"*

577

Finland has produced so many brilliant distance runners because back home it costs $2.50 a gallon for gas.

—Esa Tikkannen, Finnish pro ice-hockey forward

578

A marathon is like life with its ups and downs, but once you've done it you feel that you can do anything.

—Unknown

579

Success is peace of mind, which is a direct result of self-satisfaction in knowing you did your best to become the best that you are capable of becoming.

—John Wooden, great UCLA basketball
coach

580

You're better than you think you are and you can do more than you think you can!

—Ken Chlouber, avid marathon runner

581

One thing is for certain. Between putting on deep heating rub and going to the bathroom, you should always, always, always … wash your hands.

—Randy L. Thurman

582

Running is the classical road to self-consciousness, self-awareness, and self-reliance. Independence is the outstanding characteristic of the runner.

—Noel Carroll, Irish middle-distance
runner who set world records in the
1960s

583

A man must love a thing very much if he not only practices it without any hope of fame and money but even practices it, without any hope of doing it well.

—G. K. Chesterton, prolific English
writer, called the Prince of Paradox

584

Decide before the race the conditions that will cause you to stop and drop out. You don't want to be out there saying, "Well, gee, my leg hurts, I'm a little dehydrated, I'm sleepy, I'm tired, and it's cold and windy." And talk yourself into quitting. If you are making a decision based on how you feel at that moment, you will probably make the wrong decision.

—Dick Collins

585

Despite what seems like the extraordinary nature of these events, in the end, they make you even more human.

—Joel McNamara, author of several *for Dummies* books

586

Rewards are on a level with the effort, and the effort is extreme.

—an unidentified Utah runner from Red Fisher, a Canadian sports journalist

587

Music is my life, but running allows me to appreciate the music of the outdoors.

—Gail Williams, Associate Principal Horn, Chicago Symphony Orchestra

588

All they want to do is stop. Those that do, regret it. For those who struggle through this patch, plodding along, fueled by the deep purpose engrained in months of training, better things may lie ahead. Fat stores may kick in (there are no guarantees, but usually there is some improvement). The feeling returns that the marathon is worth the extreme effort it takes.

—Katherine Switzer and Roger Robinson in *26.2 Marathon Stories*

589

In that he didn't die at the finish line, he could have run faster.

> —Tim Noakes, a South African professor of exercise and sports science at the University of Cape Town who has run more than seventy marathons

590

Out at mile twenty-five, I feel much closer to God than I ever do in a warm and comfortable church pew.

> —William Simpson, *Marathon and Beyond*

591

All I want to do is drink beer and train like an animal.

> —Rod Dixon, winner of the 1983 NYC Marathon

592

You'll find the more difficulties you have on the way, the more you will enjoy your success.

> —Juha "the Cruel" Vaatainen, a Finnish athlete who placed first in the 5,000m and 10,000m at the 1971 European Championships

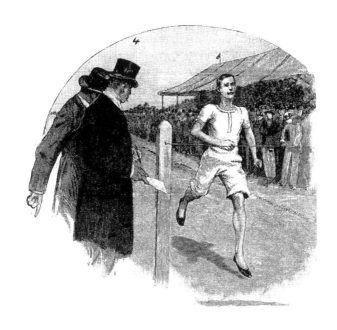

593

Whether we athletes liked it or not, the four-minute mile had become rather like an Everest: a challenge to the human spirit, it was a barrier that seemed to defy all attempts to break it, an irksome reminder that men's striving might be in vain.

—Sir Roger Bannister

594

I had no shoes and complained, until I met a man who had no feet.

—Indian Proverb

595

A man's reach must exceed his grasp, or else what's a heaven for?

—Robert Browning

596

Go fast enough to get there but slow enough to see.

—Jimmy Buffett, "Barometer Soup" lyrics

597

Racing is where I have to face the truth about myself.

—Joe Henderson, an American runner, running coach, writer, and former chief editor of *Runner's World* magazine

598

As long as you keep making RFM (relentless forward motion), you will finish.

—Stacey Page

599

For all sad words of tongue and pen, the saddest are these: "It might have been."

—John Greenleaf Whittier, an American Quaker poet, from his work *Maud Muller*

600

Dream barriers look very high until someone climbs them. They are not barriers any more.

—Lasse Viren, Finnish runner, who won gold in the 5,000m and 10,000m at the 1972 Munich Olympics

601

Now if you are going to win any battle you have to do one thing. You have to make the mind run the body. Never let the body tell the mind what to do. The body will always give up. It is always tired morning, noon, and night. But the body is never tired if the mind is not tired. When you were younger the mind could make you dance all night, and the body was never tired.… You've always got to make the mind take over and keep going.

—George S. Patton, US Army general and 1912 Olympian

602

There is the truth about the marathon and very few of you have written the truth. Even if I explain to you, you'll never understand it, you're outside of it.

—Douglas Wakiihuri, Kenyen marathon runner who won gold in the 1987 World Championships, speaking to journalists

603

I don't train to beat another runner. We are out there together, competing with the marathon, and I train to run the marathon as fast as I can.

—Juma Ikangaa, Tanzania marathon
runner

604

All our dreams can come true if we have the courage to pursue them.

—Walt Disney

605

Almost every part of the mile is tactically important: you can never let down, never stop thinking, and you can be beaten at almost any point. I suppose you could say it is like life.

—John Landy, who made a tactical error
by looking back in the final sprint in the
mile against Roger Bannister; it cost
him the race.

606

Success isn't how far you got but the distance you traveled from where you started.

—Steve Prefontaine

607

Some people can't live without booze; it looks like I can't live without running.

—Lasse Viren, Finnish long-distance
runner who won four gold Olympic
medals

608

Out of the silver heat mirage he ran. The sky burned, and under him the paving was a black mirror reflecting sun-fire. Sweat sprayed his skin with each foot strike so that he ran in a hot mist of his own creation. With each slap on the softened asphalt, his soles absorbed heat that rose through his arches and ankles and the stems of his shins. It was a carnival of pain, but he loved each stride because running distilled him to his essence and the heat hastened this distillation.

—James Tabor, from "The Runner," a
short story

609

People don't know why we run, but it's the hard work you put into practice, and the reward you get from the race.

—Courtney Parsons, runner

610

If the furnace was hot enough, anything would burn.

—Quenton Cassidy, from *Once a Runner*
by John L. Parker Jr. (sometimes
misquoted as "If the fire is hot enough,
it will burn anything")

611

I decided to go for a little run.

—Forrest Gump

612

I run because it's my passion, and not just a sport. Every
time I walk out the door, I know why I'm going where
I'm going and I'm already focused on that special place
where I find my peace and solitude. Running, to me, is
more than just a physical exercise … it's a consistent
reward for victory!

—Sasha Azevedo, American actress,
athlete, model

613

If God invented marathons to keep people from doing anything more stupid, the triathlon must have taken him completely by surprise.

—P. Z. Pearce, director of Champions
Sports Medicine in Spokane, WA

614

I believe in the runner's high, and I believe that those who are passionate about running are the ones who experience it to the fullest degree possible. To me, the runner's high is a sensational reaction to a great run! It's an exhilarating feeling of satisfaction and achievement. It's like being on top of the world, and truthfully ... there's nothing else quite like it!

—Sasha Azevedo, American actress,
athlete, model

615

Just as I always dreamed in secret, I raised my arms, I smiled, and I crossed the finish line.

—Josy Barthel, runner, 1500m, the only
athlete from Luxembourg to win a gold
Olympic medal.

616

You have brains in your head. You have feet in your shoes. You can steer yourself any direction you choose. You're on your own, and you know what you know. And you are the one who'll decide where you'll go. Oh the places you'll go.

—Dr. Suess, *Oh the Places You'll Go*

617

Every jogger can't dream of being an Olympic champion, but he can dream of finishing a marathon.

> —Fred Lebow, born in Romania, founder of the NYC Marathon. He ran in the inaugural in 1970 and ran in his last NYC Marathon in celebration of his sixtieth birthday after being diagnosed with brain cancer earlier that year. His close friend and nine-time marathon winner, Grete Waitz, ran by his side the whole way.

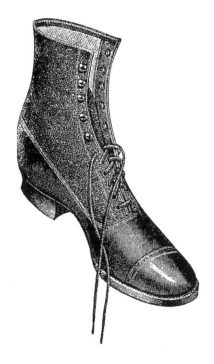

618

Nothing helps me sort out problems better than lacing up my shoes and taking a turn around the park.

—Judith Kaye, runner and former chief
judge of New York

619

If modern runners were drawn around a campfire in a warm African night, they would, like any Bushman after a hunt, poke the embers and relive the run all the way to the finish line.

—Bernd Heinrich, *Why We Run*

620

People should be encouraged to prepare properly. We need to teach them to put less emphasis on trying to perform well and more on having fun and staying within their range.

—Dr. John Bagshaw, cardiologist, giving
runners advice before a race

621

Jogging is very beneficial. It's good for your legs and your feet. It's also very good for the ground. It makes it feel needed.

—Charles Schulz, creator of the "Peanuts"
comic strip

622

Do you not know that in a race all the runners run, but only one gets the prize? Run in such a way as to get the prize.

—1 Corinthians 9:24

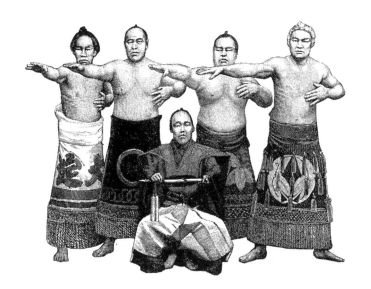

623

There is something beautiful about working so hard that you are reduced to silence next to your friends. Some friendships never get to the level where silence is comfortable, let alone productive or healing. Some friends will never understand the unspoken.

—Kristin Armstrong, author and runner

624

The starting line of the NYC Marathon is kind of a giant time bomb behind you about to go off. It is the most spectacular start in sport.

—Bill Rodgers, winner of the Boston and NYC marathons

625

I ran my first sub-four-minute mile in 1977 and since then have run 136 more. Nobody has run as many sub-fours as I have, and I intend to run at least one more.

—Steve Scott, great miler in 1995, after cancer surgery

626

In a marathon I never let myself think, *I've got 26.2 miles ahead of me.* You have to think of your race as it is then and there. At the same time you keep in mind the prospects for the future.

—Bill Rodgers, ranked number one marathon runner in the world in 1975, 1977, and 1979 by *Track and Field News*

627

I have met my hero, and he is me.

—Dr. George Sheehan, an inspirational writer on running

628

Everybody and their mother know you don't train hard on Friday, the day before a race. But a lot of runners will overtrain on Thursday if left on their own. Thursday is the most dangerous day of the week.

—Marty Stern, Villanova women's coach

629

He's fat, he's got heart disease, got diabetes—and if you don't keep running, he'll catch up with you.

—Nike

630

Just do the best with what you have, and you'll soon be doing it better.

—Gil Hodges, American Major League Baseball first baseman and manager

631

Do not let your fire go out, spark by irreplaceable spark. In the hopeless swamps of the not quite, the not yet, and the not at all, do not let the hero in your soul perish and leave only frustration for the life you deserved, but never have been able to reach. The world you desire can be won, it exists, it is real, it is possible, it is yours.

—John Galt in *Atlas Shrugged* by Ayn Rand

632

Be the change you want to see in the world.

—Mahatma Gandhi

633

So many of our dreams at first seem impossible, then they seem improbable, and then, when we summon the will, they soon become inevitable.

—Christopher Reeve (1952–2004),
American actor, director, producer,
screenwriter, and author.

634

The extra mile makes all the difference.

—Mike Pniewski, actor and dynamic
speaker on living life well

635

To succeed … you need to find something to hold on to, something to motivate you, something to inspire you.

—Tony Dorsett, Heisman Trophy winner

636

Those who say it cannot be done should not interrupt the people doing it.

—Chinese proverb

637

I laughed to myself. Here we were, no pants, and this guy is talking splits.

—Selene Yeager, fitness expert and writer
for *Runner's World*, when running in
the Bare Hare Duathlon (where you run
in the nude) and having a guy stride
with her, informing of her 6:20 pace.

638

A man can fail many times, but he isn't a failure until he begins to blame somebody else.

—Steve Prefontaine

Those Quoted

Note: numbers following entries refer to quote numbers.

Eyestone, Ed, 163

F
Faulkner, William, 27
Fixx, Jim, 26,168
Ford, Henry, 19
Fortner, Jim, 416
Foster, Charles, 332
Franklin, Barry, 132
Franklin, Benjamin, 54
Freeman, Cathy, 441

G
Galloway, Jeff, 62
Galt, John, 631
Gandhi, Mahatma, 632
Ganty, Walt, 277
Gareau, Jacqueline, 269
Garfield, 227
Gatorade ad, 92
Gerstein, Nancy, 221
Gibb, Bobbi, 365
Glover, Bob, 491
Godin, Andre, 343
Gordon, Al, 119
Graham, Martha, 331
Green, Maurice, 79
Gruber, Adolph, 165
Gump, Forrest, 229, 611
Guzzardi, Walt, 195

Index

Note: numbers following entries refer to quote
    numbers.

About the Author

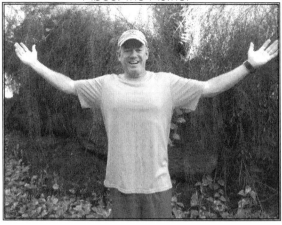

Randy L. Thurman, CPA, CFP and a runner

I am a runner, but it didn't start out that way. Turning 50 and starting to look like a pear, motivated me to do something, so I started running and haven't stopped since. It's been three years now and I am healthier, have more energy, my overall attitude improved (I could go on, see quote 126) all because of running.

In my professional life, I'm a CPA and a Certified Financial Planner™. I run a Fee-Only Investment Advisory practice in Oklahoma City, OK with 14 employees. There are many parallels to running a marathon, long-term investment success and life in general, but I will leave that for another day.

Pati, my wife, is a triathlete. I have considered doing a tri, but they won't let me in the pool with floaties on. My son Levi, is just now taking up running. I hope he will continue this lifetime sport.

91611487R00131

Made in the USA
Columbia, SC
18 March 2018